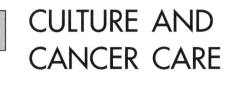

CULTURE AND CANCER CARE

FACING DEATH

Series editor: David Clark, Professor of Medical Sociology,
University of Lancaster

The subject of death in late modern culture has become a rich field of theoretical, clinical and policy interest. Widely regarded as a taboo until recent times, death now engages a growing interest among social scientists, practitioners and those responsible for the organization and delivery of human services. Indeed, how we die has become a powerful commentary on how we live, and the specialized care of dying people holds an important place within modern health and social care.

This series captures such developments. Among the contributors are leading experts in death studies, from sociology, anthropology, social psychology, ethics, nursing, medicine and pastoral care. A particular feature of the series is its attention to the developing field of palliative care, viewed from the perspectives of practitioners, planners and policy analysts; here several authors adopt a multidisciplinary approach, drawing on recent research, policy and organizational commentary, and reviews of evidence-based practice. Written in a clear, accessible style, the entire series will be essential reading for students of death, dying and bereavement, and for anyone with an involvement in palliative care research, service delivery or policy-making.

Current and forthcoming titles:

David Clark, Jo Hockley and Sam Ahmedzai (eds): *New Themes in Palliative Care*
David Clark and Jane E. Seymour: *Reflections on Palliative Care*
David Clark and Michael Wright: *Transitions in End of Life Care: Hospice and
    Related Developments in Eastern Europe and Central Asia*
Mark Cobb: *The Dying Soul: Spiritual Care at the End of Life*
Kirsten Costain Schou and Jenny Hewison: *Experiencing Cancer: Quality of Life in
    Treatment*
David Field, David Clark, Jessica Corner and Carol Davis (eds): *Researching
    Palliative Care*
Pam Firth, Gill Luff and David Oliviere: *Loss, Change and Bereavement in Palliative
    Care*
Anne Grinyer: *Cancer in Young Adults: Through Parents' Eyes*
Henk ten Have and David Clark (eds): *The Ethics of Palliative Care: European
    Perspectives*
Jenny Hockey, Jeanne Katz and Neil Small (eds): *Grief, Mourning and Death Ritual*
Jo Hockley and David Clark (eds): *Palliative Care for Older People in Care Homes*
David W. Kissane and Sidney Bloch: *Family Focused Grief Therapy*
Gordon Riches and Pam Dawson: *An Intimate Loneliness: Supporting Bereaved
    Parents and Siblings*
Lars Sandman: *A Good Death: On the Value of Death and Dying*
Jane E. Seymour: *Critical Moments: Death and Dying in Intensive Care*
Anne-Mei The: *Palliative Care and Communication: Experiences in the Clinic*
Tony Walter: *On Bereavement: The Culture of Grief*
Simon Woods: *Death's Dominion: Ethics at the End of Life*

CULTURE AND CANCER CARE

ANTHROPOLOGICAL INSIGHTS IN ONCOLOGY

SIMON DEIN

OPEN UNIVERSITY PRESS

Open University Press
McGraw-Hill Education
McGraw-Hill House
Shoppenhangers Road
Maidenhead
Berkshire
England
SL6 2QL

email: enquiries@openup.co.uk
world wide web: www.openup.co.uk

and Two Penn Plaza, New York, NY 10121-2289, USA

First published 2006

A catalogue record of this book is available from the British Library

ISBN-13:   978 0335 21458 7 (pb)   978 0335 21459 4 (hb)
ISBN-10:   0 335 21458 4 (pb)   0 335 21459 2 (hb)

Library of Congress Cataloging-in-Publication Data
CIP data applied for

Typeset by RefineCatch Ltd, Bungay, Suffolk
Printed in the UK by Bell & Bain Ltd, Glasgow

This book is dedicated to my wife, Kalpana Dein

Contents

Series editor's preface

In his classic work *The Sociological Imagination*, published in 1959, C. Wright Mills explained some of the processes whereby a phenomenon thought to be uniquely individual and personally bounded in character can come to be seen as a matter for wider concern – requiring the mobilizations of collective action and planning and thereby attracting the interests of the social analyst. Just such a transformation, from what Mills called 'private trouble' to 'public issue', is evident in the phenomenon of cancer in recent decades. For some time now, the experience of cancer has been shifting – from a disease to be endured by individual patients, with fortitude and a sense of fatalism, to become a site of wider public and professional concern as well as a specialist area for clinical attention. To understand such developments, we must examine the changing social construction of cancer as the 'dread disease' of modern culture, and move from there to an exploration of the ways in which it has been colonized by professionals, patients, policy makers and legislators. Within such a matrix, curative treatments, pain and symptom relief, and social reform are each expressed as parts of a 'cancer world' of increasing complexity and differentiation.

Causes and consequences are key dimensions in the social analysis of cancer. The former is illustrated in the proliferation of cancer and 'anti-cancer' societies since the beginnings of the twentieth century; in the rise of the oncology and radiotherapy specialisms; and in the increasing visibility of patients' experiences of cancer within public discourse and the mass media. How politics shapes what we know and do not know about cancer is an example of the second. Meanwhile, the incidence and prevalence of cancer continue to grow apace in the poorer countries of the world, and the global 'burden' of the disease is a major preoccupation for epidemiologists and strategists despite a falling public health interest in non-communicable disease.

This book by Simon Dein is an important addition to the *Facing Death* series that builds on and further develops some of these issues. It invites us to explore an anthropological perspective on cancer in which all aspects of the disease – from screening and treatment through to palliation – are consistently seen through the lens of *culture*. In a compelling introduction he lays out the importance of cancer in the contemporary world – first through a fascinating case study, then in the geographic and epidemiological contexts, before moving on to the perspectives of ethnicity, poverty and gender. A series of engrossing chapters ensues. Here Simon Dein demonstrates not only the breadth of his understanding, but also his clinical awareness and his ability to write for those who are in the frontline of service delivery. His orienting framework is that of anthropology – a discipline that has been relatively under-employed in the understanding of cancer, particularly when compared to its sister social sciences, especially psychology. Using this perspective, he begins his main analysis with a discussion of the cultural and structural factors which shape the design and uptake of screening programmes; he explores the changing practices associated with communication of the cancer diagnosis; and he examines the place of religion and spirituality in cultural and personal response to cancer. His analysis also demonstrates how cancer prognoses and outcomes vary between cultural groups; how complementary and alternative treatments gain favour; and the crucial importance of cultural issues in the delivery of palliative and end-of-life care. He concludes with an assessment of how social inequalities relating to cancer can be identified and overcome.

Culture and Cancer Care adds to several other volumes in the *Facing Death* series that focus on social, ethical and moral issues in care at the end of life and which give prominence to cultural factors. It can be read alongside ten Have and Clark's collection on the ethics of palliative care in Europe[1] and a set of writings by Ling and O'Siorain on palliative care in Ireland,[2] as well as Sandman's volume on the good death.[3] It also relates to some of the debates explored by Clark and Seymour in their sociological and policy analysis of palliative care,[4] and provides an interesting counterpoint to the factors explored by Firth and colleagues in their work on loss, change and bereavement.[5] Simon Dein has written a much needed book on the cultural aspects of cancer and it provides a valuable and welcome contribution to the *Facing Death* series.

David Clark
October 2005

References

1 ten Have, H. and Clark, D. (2002) *The Ethics of Palliative Care: European Perspectives*. Buckingham: Open University Press.
2 Ling, J. and O'Siorain, L. (eds) (2005) *Palliative Care in Ireland*. Maidenhead: Open University Press.
3 Sandman, L. (2005) A *Good Death*. Maidenhead: Open University Press.
4 Clark, D. and Seymour, J. (1999) *Reflections on Palliative Care*. Buckingham: Open University Press.
5 Firth, P., Luff, G. and Oliviere, D. (2005) *Loss, Change and Bereavement in Palliative Care*. Maidenhead: Open University Press.

Acknowledgements

I wish to thank personally Professor Roland Littlewood, Dr Cecil Helman, Dr Maurice Lipsedge, Professor David Napier, Dr Kalpana Dein, Dr Subia Rushid, Dr Alex Gath and Professor Deborah Gordon who have read earlier manuscripts of my book. This book builds on an earlier paper: Dein, S. (2004a) Explanatory models and attitudes towards cancer in different cultures, *The Lancet Oncology* 5:119–24 (Elsevier Science). Some of the material in this book has appeared in: Dein, S. and Thomas, K. (2002) To tell or not to tell: cultural and religious factors related to the disclosure of a fatal prognosis, *European Journal of Palliative Care* 9(5): 209–12 (Hayward Medical); Dein, S. (2003) Mind-body therapies and the psycho-oncology debate, *European Journal of Palliative Care* 103: 30–2 (Hayward Medical); Dein, S. (2004) From chaos to cosmogeny: a comparison of understandings of the narrative process among Western academics and Hasidic Jews, *Anthropology and Medicine* 11(2): 135–47 (Taylor and Francis Publishers); Dein, S. (2005) Attitudes towards cancer among elderly Bangladeshis in London, *European Journal of Cancer Care* (Blackwell Publishing); Dein, S. (in press) Culture and delay in help seeking for breast cancer: what are the implications for health communication? *International Journal of Cancer Prevention* (Nova Publishers); Dein, S. and Bhui, K. (in preparation) Informed consent for medical research among non-westernised ethnic minority patients: a discussion paper, *Journal of Royal Society of Medicine* (The Royal Society of Medicine); Dein, S. (in preparation) Race, culture and ethnicity in ethnic minority research: a critical discussion, *Journal of Cultural Diversity* (Tucker Publications). I am grateful for permission from these publishers to reproduce some of these ideas (in content).

In particular, two recent comprehensive reviews of the area have stimulated my thinking about this topic: Ward, E., Jemal, A., Cokkinides, V. *et al.*

(2004) Cancer disparities by race / ethnicity and socio-economic status, *CA: A Cancer Journal for Clinicians*, 54: 78–93, and Freeman, H. (2004) Poverty, culture and social injustice: cancer disparities, *Cancer Journal Clinics*, 54: 72–7. I would like to thank these authors. Lastly, I am grateful to Professor J. Kai for his excellent book *Ethnicity, Health and Primary Care*, (2003) which has facilitated my discussion of cross-cultural communication.

The details of the case studies presented in the book, although taken from clinical practice, have been changed substantially to maintain confidentiality. All the views expressed in this book are my own.

Introduction

Salma had only been living in the UK for five years when she developed colorectal cancer. Following the death of her husband in Pakistan, she had emigrated to live with her daughter Moona, her daughter's husband Tariq and their four children. The family lived in a two bedroom overcrowded house on a run down housing estate in the North of England. She spoke and understood English very poorly. She seldom left her house and, on account of this, she mixed very little with anyone outside her own cultural group.

The diagnosis of cancer came as a shock to Salma's family. She had consulted her general practitioner on numerous occasions with abdominal pain, only to be told it was constipation and that it would resolve itself. When she was referred to the hospital, it was as an emergency, and she required urgent surgery. Her consultant was unable to communicate with her directly, and explained her 'serious diagnosis' to her family, hoping that they would translate for him. This, however, did not go smoothly. Her son-in-law asked the consultant not to disclose the fact that she had cancer to her, since in Pakistan it was common for relatives, not the patients themselves, to be given the diagnosis. The consultant was not happy to withhold this information from her and explained that she had every right to know her diagnosis. Finally, and very reluctantly, another family member explained to her that she had cancer. Rather surprisingly she seemed to accept the diagnosis very well although it was uncertain how much she really understood about the illness. Salma had always been a devout Muslim who believed strongly that her destiny was in God's hands and that whatever happened would be for the best. She was comforted by regular visits from a local imam and by her frequent prayers which gave her a sense of calm.

Her initial treatment with chemotherapy went well. She seemed to regain some strength and was able to get about by herself for a couple of months.

But the improvement was not long lasting. She slowly became weaker, lost her appetite and vomited frequently. Further investigations revealed that her cancer had spread to her liver. Both she and her family refused further chemotherapy but were happy to accept strong painkillers. In the hope that she might be cured, her son-in-law contacted a healer in Pakistan who recited passages from the Qur'an, prepared a *taveez* (amulet) and recommended that she drank holy water.

Her deterioration continued. After a couple of weeks she required admission to her local hospice. While there, several 'problems' arose. Following an episode where she refused to undress to be examined by a male doctor, the nurses asked why she was being 'difficult'. Her admission was during the fast of Ramadan, a time when Muslims are expected to fast during the daylight hours. Although she herself chose not to eat during the day, there were several 'concerns' expressed by hospice staff about her poor food intake which was attributed to her illness. Lastly, the family felt upset since there was no private room in which they could pray. She died two weeks later. Following her death the nurses were concerned about how they should treat the body. They commented that they had never looked after a devout Muslim patient before.

The case study above illustrates a number of points related to Salma's culture: the role of the family in medical decision making; her appeal to religion as a way of coping; the use of traditional healing alongside biomedicine; her poor understanding of English; the emphasis on modesty; the importance of religious festivals; and finally a lack of medical staff knowledge about the rites of death and dying in Islam. These occurred against the background of socio-economic deprivation and poor (in this case significantly delayed) medical care. Obvious conflicts related to cultural differences are apparent.

It is important to avoid the pitfalls of cultural stereotyping, seeing ethnic minority groups as homogeneous entities, with all those belonging to a specific group holding the same beliefs and behaving in the same way when faced with similar life situations. Some members of ethnic minority groups continue to live a traditional way of life, differing little from that in their country of origin. Others have adapted to the way of life of the majority group, and have adopted its values. For these people, traditional cultural beliefs only come to the fore at certain times. For everyone, however, serious life-threatening illness, such as cancer, requires more than explanation; it requires a framework which can be used to re-establish meaning in a world shattered by illness. This framework is provided by culture and religion.

Cancer is more than a biological disease. Cultural factors are involved at every stage in the journey through cancer, from prevention to palliative care. Even the definition of what constitutes cancer varies according to the cultural context. A study among African American women with breast and cervical cancer in Atlanta elicited the belief that the only real cancer was a late stage cancer causing death and that a non-fatal condition could not be cancer and therefore screening was of little use. For this group cancer was held to be incurable and ultimately the women believed that their destinies were determined by God. The most common explanations for cancer included a bruise or a sore that would not heal. Moreover, they held that the knowledge that one had early cancer could cause mental distress which could possibly speed up death (Gregg and Curry 1994).

In some societies there is in fact no word for cancer (Kaur 1996). Bezwoda *et al.* (1997) point out that in only three of the nine ethnic Black languages in South Africa (Zulu, Swazi and Xhosa) is there a word for cancer at all. These words do not refer to a disease that could spread to other parts of the body or requires any specific treatments to bring about cure. In Nigeria there is no common name for cancer among traditional healers. In some groups there may be several local terms connoting various types of cancer at various locations of the body.

The experience of illness cannot be considered in isolation from the cultural context in which it occurs. This is especially the case for life-threatening illnesses such as cancer where issues of meaning become paramount. Social attitudes towards cancer, how it is understood, participation in screening, health behaviour, treatments used and palliative care vary significantly across cultures. Issues related to the communication of the diagnosis and decisions about treatment (and the ethics of treating or withholding treatment) are highly variable across cultural groups. These issues in turn are related to broader ideas of autonomy, personal control (and its opposite, fatalism), explanatory models, attributional styles, ideas of personhood (including the mind-body distinction) and ultimate concerns about life and death in a given society – something that might be called spirituality.

Cancer in contemporary Western culture

Despite recent advances in the treatment of cancer, this disease remains a major world killer. The very word strikes a chord of terror in those who suffer from it. Patterson (1987) in *The Dread Disease: Cancer and Modern American Culture* points out the contemporary deep-seated fear concerning cancer in contemporary American culture, a fear which emerged during the second half of the nineteenth century. Although about 50 per cent of cases of cancer are potentially curable, lay people in both Western and non-Western cultures still have a universal dread of cancer. In most instances the disease remains highly stigmatized.

Although there is a large literature examining the causes, symptoms and treatments of this disease, there is relatively little work which looks at how attitudes, understandings and responses to cancer vary across cultures. The contemporary literature on cancer can be divided into three types: biomedical; self-help books including those on complementary and alternative medicine; and first hand accounts of cancer by sufferers themselves. There are many books written by authors grounded in a biomedical tradition discussing the facts about the various types of cancer and their treatments (by radiotherapy, chemotherapy and surgery). These are useful for cancer patients who want biomedical information about their cancer. Books about complementary and alternative treatments for cancer appear to be flourishing (e.g. Hay 1989; Siegel 1993). Much of the market is monopolized by the so-called 'self-help' books, offering advice about coping with the disease and how complementary or alternative therapies can be helpful. Often these books talk of overcoming cancer through willpower or major lifestyle changes.

Since the mid-1990s there has been a new genre of writing – books written by patients and their relatives about the experience of cancer. Some of these, such as *Teratologies* (Stacey 1997); *The Wounded Storyteller* (Frank 1995); and the recent *Stranger in the Village of the Sick: A Memoir of Cancer, Sorcery and Healing* (Stoller 2004) are written by social scientists who happen to have cancer themselves and discuss contemporary cultural and anthropological themes while describing their individual experiences of cancer. They provide a critique of Western biomedicine's conceptualization of the body as separate from the self or person, whereby the patient's illness is reduced to a 'case' that can be quantified in terms of its symptoms and modes of treatment.

Although *Culture and Cancer Care* is exemplified by individual case studies, much of the information presented below is epidemiological, using data from the literature which examines the relationship between cultural factors and various types of cancer across a number of cultural groups. Unlike other recent books which have focused on cultural aspects of cancer (e.g. Moore and Spiegel, 2004, *Cancer, Culture and Communication*, which emphasizes how cultural contexts influence cancer communication), this book integrates anthropological ideas into oncology and is as much a critique of essentialist notions such as culture, race and ethnicity in the oncology field. A central theme of this book is to discuss cancer inequalities in relation to the unequal distribution of power and resources within societies and its relationship to wider social issues such as racism. As such, it deploys a political economy approach – one that emphasizes the consequences of power and resources for health and mortality.

Geographical focus

The literature discussed in this book derives from North America, Canada, the United Kingdom, Europe and Australia although the majority of studies quoted are from the UK and USA. Despite the fact that the demographic structures of the UK and USA are different, both have racial and ethnic minority populations who have poorer health than the general population, including increased rates of some types of cancer and poorer prognoses.

There are significant differences between the healthcare systems in the latter two countries, which influence how cancer patients are treated and the eventual outcome. In the USA there is a liberal healthcare system whereby the majority of the citizens have obtained healthcare by their own means, especially by subscribing to private insurance. Coverage is usually employer based, although 40–50 per cent of the funding derives from government programmes such as Medicare or Medicaid. Many people in this situation are not insured or are underinsured (about 44 million people) and are denied high quality medical care. Speciality and tertiary care dominate the US system, which is highly influenced by the principles of entrepreneurship and the free market economy.

The American situation is to be contrasted with the British state-run system of healthcare, whereby its cost is paid for out of taxes and is free at point of use for British citizens and those from the EEC. Healthcare is seen as a public service and coverage is universal. In the UK system there is an emphasis on primary care providers (General Practitioners or GPs) at the point of access. The role of private providers is limited. These different systems significantly influence access and quality of cancer healthcare among different sectors of the population.

What is cancer and what causes it?

Cancer is the disordered and uncontrolled growth of cells within a specific organ or tissue type. Most cancers begin in a single site such as breast, lung or bowel. If untreated the cancer grows and can invade normal tissues causing extensive tissue destruction with resulting functional damage. It may also spread through the blood stream and lymphatic system to produce secondary growths termed metastases. These may themselves cause profound damage and are often life threatening. We are still ignorant of the mechanisms causing metastases.

Factors known from epidemiological studies to be causally related to the development of cancer include environmental factors such as smoking (lung, larynx, pancreas, mouth, kidney and bladder) and diet (fat intake and breast cancer). Other environmental factors derive from working in specific occupations (e.g. dye workers and bladder cancers, asbestos workers and mesothelioma). Age is a major risk factor for many cancers (lung, oesophagus, stomach, pancreas, prostate, breast and uterine). Greater age at first pregnancy has been shown to increase the risk of breast cancer. Up to 10 per cent of common cancers, particularly those of breast, ovary and large bowel, occur in familial clusters and are related to a familial gene. There is some evidence that viral infections may cause cancer (nasopharyngeal cancer in China and the Epstein Barr virus, papilloma virus and cervical cancer). Radiation may be responsible for the development of thyroid, leukaemia, lymphoma and lung cancer. Souhami and Tobias (2002) have provided an excellent overview of this area.

A major public health problem

According to the World Health Organisation (Lopez 1990; World Health Organisation 1991), in 1985 nearly 50 million people died worldwide. Cancer was the cause of 10 per cent of deaths, 23 per cent died of circulatory diseases and 5 per cent died of chronic obstructive lung diseases. The largest proportion of deaths were caused by infectious and parasitic diseases (36 per cent). However this situation is likely to change rapidly with progress in treating infectious diseases. A projection of mortality and the causes of death indicate that in 2015 the major causes of death will relate to non-communicable diseases. It is estimated that cancer and circulatory diseases will account for 54 per cent of all deaths in this year (Bulatao and Stephens 1991). The major increases will occur in developing countries. These figures do not take into account the large numbers of AIDS sufferers of whom between 10–40 per cent develop malignant tumours.

Lung cancer and AIDS are already major causes of death worldwide and it is likely that these two diseases will continue to be major killers in the early part of the twenty-first century (Lopez 1990; World Health Organisation 1991). Lung cancer is emerging as a major health problem in many developing countries, especially Africa, and is the most frequent cancer worldwide (Parkin et al. 1988; Ferlay et al. 2004). This is as a result of increasing tobacco use. Although potentially preventable and dependent on lifestyle, high mortality rates spread from industrialized countries to the rest of the world. This disease is essentially incurable and major resources will be required to adequately palliate its symptoms. Of the estimated 10 million tobacco related deaths in the year 2015, about three million are expected to occur in China alone and almost one million of these deaths will be from lung cancer (Stjernsward and Clark 2003).

Approximately 60 per cent of the world's new cancer patients occur in developing countries and at least 80 per cent of these are incurable at the time of diagnosis. These figures have implications for both resources and treatments. About 75 per cent of total healthcare spending, public and private, in developing countries goes on curative efforts mainly in hospitals which are located in urban areas, despite the fact that most of the population resides in rural areas. There is a need for a comprehensive approach to the development of a coherent prevention, treatment and care policy for those with cancer and AIDS related cancer, with perhaps greater emphasis being given to prevention and palliative care rather than curative efforts. These trends are of great interest and significance in themselves, and will provide much needed data for cancer epidemiologists and health providers. In this book however the focus is on cancer in developed countries.

The epidemiology of cancer in the USA and UK

Epidemiology is the study of the distribution, determinants and frequency of disease in human populations. Epidemiologists use a number of terms to describe rates of illness. The term 'incidence' refers to the number of new cases of illness which occur in a population in a defined time period. It is usually expressed as a percentage, or as a number of cases per 1000 or per 100,000 people in the population. The term 'prevalence' refers to the total number of existing cases of a disease at that time divided by the number of the population at risk.

Cancer is a common disease in the UK. As a cause of mortality it is second only to cardiovascular disease. It is the cause of 26 per cent of all deaths in the UK (Office for National Statistics 2002) and is diagnosed each year in one in 250 men and one in every 300 women. Over the age of 60, three in every 100 men develop the disease each year (Souhami and Tobias 1998). Approximately one in three people will develop cancer in their lifetime (Cancer Research UK 2004).

One in four deaths in the United States is attributable to cancer, and one in three Americans will eventually develop some form of cancer (Haynes and Smedley 1999). One half of new cases of cancer occur in people aged 65 years and over (US Department of Health and Human Services 2000). In 1999 cancer accounted for 440, 000 deaths among older persons in the USA and is now the leading cause of death for Americans aged 60–79 years, and the second leading cause of death for those over 80 years (Jemal *et al.* 2002). A collaborative report between the American Cancer Society, the National Cancer Institute, the National Institute on Aging and the Centers for Disease Control and Prevention (Edwards *et al.* 2002) notes that cancer has surpassed heart disease as the major killer of Americans under the age of 85 years and that it accounts for one in every four deaths. The report estimates that the total number of cancer cases can be expected to double by 2050 if current incidence rates remain stable on account of the ageing structure of the US population.

Cancer in ethnic minority groups in the USA

According to the latest estimates, roughly one in every three people in the United States belongs to a racial and ethnic minority group. Latinos (the largest racial and ethnic minority group) and African Americans together account for 25 per cent of the total US population. In the next 50 years, the proportions of both Latinos and Asian Americans/Pacific Islanders are expected to double (US Bureau of the Census, Census 2000). Despite improved understandings of cancer control, prevention, detection and treatment, not all segments of the US population have benefited from the advances in the understanding of cancer.

Although many ethnic minority groups experience significantly lower levels of some types of cancer than the general population, for other groups, the incidence and mortality rates are significantly higher. Black American males are more likely to develop cancer than other ethnic groups and are about 33 per cent more likely to die of cancer than White Americans (American Cancer Society 2000; NCI 2002; Ries *et al.* 2003, 2004). This disparity in death rates from all cancers combined between African American and White males widened from 1975 until the early 1990s. The gap has subsequently narrowed but remains larger than it did in 1975. Similar, but less marked, trends have been observed between African American women and White women (Mariotto *et al.* 2002; Ward *et al.* 2004).

During the period 1992–1998, the average annual incidence rate for all cancer sites was 445.3 per 100,000 persons among Black people, 401.4 per 100,000 among White people, 283.4 per 100,000 for Asian/Pacific Islanders, 270.0 per 100,000 among Hispanics, and 202.7 per 100,000 among American Indians/Native Alaskans. Black American men have the highest incidence rates of prostate, colon, rectum, lung and bronchus cancers and are 75 per cent more likely to develop prostate cancer than other groups in the USA (Garfinkel and Mushinski 1999).

Incidence rates of lung cancer among Black men in the USA are about 50 per cent higher than in White men (110.7 versus 72.6 per 100,000). Native Hawaiian men also have elevated rates of lung cancer compared to White men. Alaskan men and women suffer disproportionately higher rates of cancer of the colon and rectum than White people. Vietnamese women in the United States have a higher cervical cancer incidence rate, more than five times greater than White women (Ries *et al.* 2004). Hispanic women also suffer elevated rates of cervical cancer. An increasingly large consistent body of research indicates that racial and ethnic minorities in the USA are less likely to receive even routine medical procedures and experience a lower quality of health services (Geiger 2001; Rutledge 2001).

Cancer in ethnic minorities in the UK

Ethnic minorities constitute 6 per cent of the total population in the UK and Wales; just under a half are from the Indian subcontinent, one third are Afro-Caribbean or African and 5 per cent are Chinese. A major problem in establishing cancer epidemiology in the UK is a lack of relevant data on ethnicity. There is some data suggesting that mortality from cancer among ethnic minorities is lower than for the White majority. However this research relates to migrants rather than those born in England and Wales (Bhal 1996). Nonetheless cancer still remains a major source of mortality in this group (Bhopal and Rankin 1996). The cancer mortality is likely to increase as the mean age of this population increases and certain lifestyle and environmental factors are increasingly acquired (Bhal 1996).

To date there have been few studies of cancer incidence by ethnic group in the UK. The most comprehensive evidence is that reported by Harding and Rosato (1999) based on a survey of Scottish, Irish, West Indian and South Asian migrants in England and Wales. The incidence of all malignant neoplasms was low among West Indians and Indians and this pattern was consistent among South Asians for Hindus, Sikhs and Muslims. A low incidence of breast cancer was found in West Indian and South Asian females. The study concluded that, although the risks of the main cancers were lower among West Indians and South Asians compared to the general population, they were still a cause for concern. Breast cancer was the commonest cancer in all migrant female groups and lung cancer was the commonest cancer in migrant male groups.

Unlike in the USA, there is to date relatively little research which has focused upon access to treatment for ethnic minority cancer sufferers in the UK. There have been no comprehensive studies of equity of access to cancer services for minority ethnic groups. However, the third national survey of NHS cancer patients suggests many areas of disadvantage. This study was designed to monitor the NHS performance as seen from the patient's perspective (Department of Health 2004).

Epidemiological studies point to the fact that some rare forms of cancer occur almost exclusively in specific ethnic minority groups in the UK and USA. These include

1 Oropharyngeal cancer in South Asians, especially Bangladeshis, because of beetle nut chewing (Balarajan and Bulusu 1990);
2 Hepatoma in South East Asians, Middle Eastern and African people and South Asian and Caribbean men (linked to infection with Hepatitis B, C and alcohol; Balarajan and Bulusu 1990);
3 Nasopharyngeal cancer in South East Asians;
4 Stomach cancer in South East Asians.

Cancer and poverty

It appears that some types of cancer and poorer prognoses are more prevalent in certain ethnic groups. It is not just ethnic minorities who have increased rates of some types of cancer. Individuals of all ethnic backgrounds who are poor, lack health insurance, or have inadequate access to high quality cancer care experience high cancer incidence and mortality rates and low rates of survival from the disease (American Cancer Society 1989). It has been repeatedly shown that the highest rates of poverty are concentrated among the same subgroups with disproportionately worse health status both in the UK and in the USA (Nazroo and Davey-Smith 2001). Poverty may increase rates of cancer through its influence on lifestyle or by negatively influencing access to treatments, a phenomenon which may be intensified by racist attitudes of health professionals and the wider society. Cancer disparities are driven by a complex interrelating set of social, economic, cultural and health system factors (Haynes and Smedley 1999; Freeman 2004).

However, it must be emphasized that cancer is *both* a disease of poverty and a disease of affluence. Affluence elevates cancer risk both in individuals and nations possibly through its influence on diet (high fat content and overeating) and lifestyle. For example, breast cancer has typically been portrayed as a 'disease of affluence' and has been linked to levels of economic development. Although this cancer has been more common in industrialized, affluent countries and among more affluent women in any given country, incidence rates in poorer countries and among poorer women in more affluent countries are slowly catching up (Stoll 1996; Stoll 2000; Hall and Rockhill 2002).

A brief note on gender

There is an emerging literature suggesting that there are striking differences in mortality and illness between men and women in industrialized societies. Within ethnic minority groups, gender may play a significant role in determining the experience of cancer, death and dying. However, to date, the topic of gender has been neglected in the literature about modern death, dying and bereavement, with authors assuming that there are no significant gender differences. There are however some important exceptions (Bronfen 1992; Cline 1995). In relation to cancer, Klonoff and Landrine (1994) looked at how males and females attributed cause to six illnesses: AIDS, diabetes mellitus, the common cold, hypertension, lung cancer and headaches. The causal attributions were found to be more complex than those in the existing literature. Although there were no differences between minorities and White people in the perceived causes of illness, men were significantly less likely than women to view illness as caused by sin, sex or as a form of punishment. This study underscores the importance of moving beyond ethnicity to examine gender differences in the perception of illness causation. The topic of gender will not be further explored here. For a good overview of the ways in which gender shapes the experience of dying and bereavement see Field *et al.* (1997).

Themes in the book

This book concentrates on three main themes. First, disparities in incidence and mortality rates of cancer in different ethnic groups are examined in relation to cultural beliefs, socio-economic status (including poverty) and racism. A critical approach is taken towards the notion of culture, moving beyond the naïve idea that it is a fixed set of beliefs held by a group of people, to a notion of culture as a dynamic framework for interpreting and understanding the world, which closely interrelates with wider social issues including racism and deprivation.

Second, ideas about sickness and help-seeking behaviour must be understood in their cultural context. How people understand cancer and what they do about it vary across cultural groups and are closely related to wider views about suffering and misfortune and conceptualizations about agency, responsibility and autonomy.

Third, in contemporary Western culture, although biomedicine has made significant advances in the treatment of some types of cancer, many sufferers and their families have become disillusioned with the biomedical reductionism and its emphasis on disease rather than illness. There has been increasing recourse to complementary and alternative medicines (CAM) over the past twenty years. The cultural issues to this phenomenon make up a third theme of this book.

Book outline

Each chapter focuses on a specific area of cancer care:

1 The relevance of anthropology

This chapter introduces key ethnographic terms: culture, race, ethnicity, disease and illness. It discusses the problems with culturalist explanations of illness and emphasizes the importance of socio-economic factors, unequal distribution of power and resources in disparities in health and illness. It moves on to look at explanatory models of cancer and qualitative research followed by a discussion of a number of anthropological themes: self, autonomy, narrative, metaphors of illness and the expression of emotion.

2 Screening and cancer prevention across cultures: moving beyond culture

Studies in the USA and UK indicate that some ethnic groups have poor uptakes for screening and the possible explanations for this are discussed: lack of knowledge and understanding of screening in some groups; fatalistic attitudes towards cancer; and economic factors, such as lack of financial resources. The chapter ends by discussing ways in which rates of screening can be improved and the role of culturally sensitive health education in this process.

3 Communicating the diagnosis and cancer communication

There are variations in the way that a diagnosis of cancer is communicated. In many non-Western cultures it is the family who are told about the diagnosis, not the patient. This can cause major problems working with such patients in Western settings where the ethos is towards open disclosure. These trends are changing in many parts of the world. The Anglo-American approach of disclosure differs from the norm in many other cultures, where the diagnosis is withheld to prevent loss of hope. But what is hope and how does it vary cross-culturally? The relationship between disclosure and the ethics of autonomy are discussed.

4 The cultural response to cancer, coping and the role of religion and spirituality

Medical anthropological studies indicate that the expression of emotion is influenced by culture. There are strong social conventions which permit or prohibit the public expression of emotion. In some cultures anger is a common response to a diagnosis of cancer, whereas in other cultures the expression of anger is seen as lack of faith in God. The communication of cancer pain is highly variable across cultures and can vary from crying to stoicism. Similarly, patients' relatives express emotions differently in different cultures. It is important for professionals working with patients from other cultures to understand modes of emotional expression so that they are not labelled as 'unacceptable' or 'pathological'. Various forms of coping with cancer are discussed, leading to a consideration of the role of religion and spirituality in the coping process.

5 Culture, cancer and treatment

There is substantial evidence that the prognoses for some cancers are worse in some cultural groups. The possible reasons for this are discussed: late presentation; lack of treatment; non-compliance with treatment; the use of traditional healing; and racist attitudes among healthcare professionals. Biological explanations of this phenomenon are critiqued. The chapter ends with a consideration of delays in help seeking for breast cancer among various ethnic groups, emphasizing the role of cultural beliefs and the family in medical decision making.

6 Complementary and alternative therapies in oncology

Complementary and alternative therapies are becoming increasingly popular in the treatment of cancer. What socio-cultural factors are responsible for this? This increasing popularity is discussed in relation to disillusionment with conventional treatments, the consumerist ethic, issues of control and the lack of perceived holism of conventional treatments.

7 Cultural aspects of palliative care, death and dying

Cultural factors significantly impact on the experience of death and dying. Attitudes to a good and bad death vary across cultural groups, as do beliefs about where and how the person should die. In many cultures the process of death and dying is highly ritualized and these rituals facilitate the rite of passage for the patient and his or her family. Spiritual beliefs relating to the meaning of life and death and notions of an afterlife are closely tied to the experience of dying. The importance of prayer, diet and religious personnel in the care of the dying is discussed in relation to a number of religious groups. This chapter includes a section on cultural aspects of bereavement.

8 Tackling inequalities in cancer outcomes

Reducing inequalities in cancer treatments and outcomes may be addressed at a number of levels, both nationally (through political and legal manoeuvres) and at the local level through community health education interventions. These interventions must go beyond changing 'inappropriate' cultural beliefs to addressing issues of racism and discrimination. Issues related to access to cancer diagnosis and treatments are discussed. The importance of developing cultural competence for health professionals is underscored. This chapter emphasizes the role of community health educators (CHE) in carrying out these health interventions in their local communities.

Further reading

Bartley, M., Blane, D. and Davey Smith, G. (eds) (1998) *Sociology of Health Inequalities*. Sociology of Health and Illness Monograph. Oxford: Blackwell Publishers.

Haynes, M. and Smedley, B. (1999) *The Unequal Burden of Cancer: An Assessment of NIH Research and Programs for Ethnic Minorities and the Medically Underserved*. Washington DC: National Academy Press.

Singer, M. and Baer, H. (1995) *Critical Medical Anthropology*. Amityville, NY: Baywood Press.

Souhami, R. and Tobias, G. (1998) *Cancer and its Management*. London: Blackwell.

1 The relevance of anthropology

Anthropology is the study of mankind in its widest context. The field can be divided into archaeology (the investigation of human cultures of the past through the recovery of material remains), material culture (man's material environment), and social anthropology (the study of man's social environment including institutions such as kinship, economics, marriage and religion). Medical anthropology is a branch of social anthropology and refers to the study of social and cultural dimensions of health, sickness and medicine. This book specifically addresses medical anthropological issues. However, the field of oncology cannot ignore the findings of archaeology, which indicate that cancer is indeed found in ancient civilizations (Roberts and Manchester 2001). Although we are limited by the fact that all that remains of ancient bodies are the skeletons (apart from rare mummified specimens), it appears that diseases such as osteosarcoma and multiple myeloma existed in early societies. For instance, a humerus from Iron-Age Switzerland displaying the pathological findings of osteosarcoma and evidence of multiple myeloma was found in an adult female skull in Caudiville, Peru dating back to 500 AD.

Medical anthropology has developed significantly since the 1980s, with anthropologists taking a particular interest in the specific domain of sickness. Anthropological approaches emphasize three main tenets: first, anthropology emphasizes holism. This is the idea that any social institution cannot be understood in isolation. Each social institution interrelates with other social institutions. For example, sickness can only be understood by taking into account ideas about kinship, economics and religion and is related to wider concepts of autonomy, the self and misfortune in general. Helman (2001: 50) states how 'Anthropologists have pointed out that any society's healthcare system cannot be studied in isolation from other aspects of that society, especially its social, religious, political and economic organisation.'

Second is the idea of relativism. Each cultural group has their own specific ways of understanding a cultural phenomenon. We must learn to understand sickness from their own point of view and move away from ethnocentrism (seeing something from our own culture's perspective). Even biomedical knowledge, the dominant medical system in Western cultures based on scientific rational empiricism, itself is culturally constructed. Despite the fact that biomedicine claims to be universal, various studies point to the fact that there are significant differences in the types of diagnoses given and the treatments prescribed between different Western medical systems. Terms such as 'family', 'religion' and 'medicine' may have specific meanings for cultures and cannot be taken for granted. Understandings of specific diseases such as cancer cannot be divorced from the wider cultural perspective in which suffering is understood.

Third, beliefs may not reflect actions. Ideas about treating illness and lay explanatory models are shaped by contingent circumstances and forms of practical 'reasoning in action' (Lambert and McKevitt 2002). A person may believe one thing and do another. Medical anthropologists are interested not just in what people say about sickness but what they actually do in practice. Methodologically, there is an emphasis on participant observation – direct observation while participating in a study community. Medical anthropologists observe real life scenarios of healing and in the process attempt to understand how groups of people engage in medical decision making. This is directly relevant to oncology. For instance, women may state specific negative beliefs about screening for cancer yet still partake in the screening process. A medical anthropologist would attempt to explain this discrepancy.

A number of themes are commonly discussed in contemporary medical and psychiatric anthropology: disease and illness; health, culture and ethnicity; the political economy of health; explanatory models; metaphors of illness; the self and agency; narratives; and the cultural construction of emotion. These are discussed below, beginning with the distinction between disease and illness.

Disease and illness

Medical anthropologists make a distinction between disease and illness (Kleinman 1990). The former refers to pathology in the cells, tissues and organs. The latter refers to the social and psychological response to the underlying disease and also the ways in which it is conceptualized and understood. The two are different. This book focuses on illness. The social and psychological response to cancer and the ways in which it is understood are influenced by the cultural context. It is possible to have a disease without illness. For example, a person may be 'harbouring' an early cancer and not have any symptoms. The finding of early asymptomatic cancer is the aim of cancer screening. On the other hand, the person may have a belief that they have cancer but there is no cancer found. This person has an illness but not a disease.

Culture, race and ethnicity and anti-racism

Culture, race and ethnicity are terms commonly used in the health literature, often in confusing and contradictory ways. The term 'culture' is probably the most commonly used concept in anthropology, although there is much debate as to the exact meaning of the term. Definitions of culture vary in emphasis between the humanistic – culture is what a person ought to acquire in order to become a fully worthwhile moral agent – and the anthropological sense in which the world is divided into different cultures each with its own worth. Each particular person is a product of a particular culture.

The term must be distinguished from race: a framework of ranked categories based on biological characteristics which divide up human populations and society. This concept was formulated in a time of social Darwinism and is now discredited as a biological descriptor. The term has been attacked and undermined by advances in genetics. In contemporary writings the term race is virtually indistinguishable from ethnicity and the concept of race is slowly being redefined as a cultural and socio-political construct. Despite much theoretical critique, many researchers have been convinced of the continuing potential of the term to explain genetic differences in rates of some diseases such as hypertension (Baker *et al.* 1998).

In much of the research addressing health inequalities, colour may be an important indicator of historical and current discrimination. However, health inequality is likely to be a result of social factors including poverty, diet, employment, etc. Only for a few specific genetic diseases will biological factors be important causes. The example of the haemoglobinopathies such as sickle cell disease may be cited here. The role of biology has far too often been implicated as an explanation for racial differences in disease rates.

Another term commonly used in the literature is 'ethnicity'. The term is neither simple nor precise but implies one or more of the following: shared origins or social background, shared culture, and traditions that are distinctive, maintained between generations and lead to a sense of group identity and common language or religious tradition (Senior and Bhopal 1994). It emphasizes shared history, geographical origins, language, diet and other features.

A large social anthropological and sociological literature exists about ethnicity and there is little consensus about the categorization of ethnicities. Macbeth (2001) argues that accurate definitions of ethnic groups are impossible on account of the absence of meaningful boundaries but nevertheless some factors which can be called ethnic are highly significant to health experience. For second generation people who were born and educated in the UK and have British accents, the ethnicity definition is very problematic. For the same individual, different ethnic identities come into play at different times and in different contexts. The term is not politically neutral and can serve a similar function to race in the portrayal of cultural difference as deviant or pathological. There is thus a continuing need for the concepts of race and ethnicity to be strictly demarcated and used precisely. One possible advance as Bhopal (2001) argues is to replace the terms race and ethnicity with the term 'identifiable populations'.

The ethnic terms 'White', 'Black' and 'Asian' are commonly used in the UK, whereas 'White', 'Black' and 'Hispanic' are used in American articles. The term Asian in the USA refers to Chinese and Japanese whereas in the UK it refers to those from the Indian subcontinent. From April 1995 the British Department of Health has required hospitals to collect data on the ethnicity of patients and has deployed categories based on census data. This in turn may help to further understand the often complex relationships between ethnicity and cancer incidences and mortality.

Over time, members of ethnic minority groups may learn to become a member of the host culture, a process referred to as acculturation. The term is commonly used in the health literature, although it is seen by anthropologists and sociologists as being an outdated concept which has undesirable connotations. Some degree of acculturation may in fact occur prior to emigration. In the past the assumption was held that those who did not change to majority cultural values were being 'inconvenient'. The term does not allow for the change which the majority culture undergoes through contact with minority cultures. Following immigration, ethnic minorities may in fact more strongly adhere to their traditional cultural practices to maintain their self identities and this may occur especially at times of serious illness such as cancer.

Within any ethnic minority group, levels of acculturation in relation to health and illness may differ in terms of fluency in the national language and how au-fait an individual is with the majority culture's conceptualizations of health, illness and healing. As Ahmad (1993) notes, there is a difference between being aware of the health beliefs of another culture and actually sharing these beliefs. For example, a member of an ethnic minority group may speak English fluently and adopt certain practices of the majority culture, but refer to the beliefs of their ethnic group when conceptualizing health. In the UK some ethnic minority communities may maintain distinctive definitions of illness and traditions of healthcare (Bhopal 1986; Krause 1989). Their health beliefs and knowledge may be incongruent with that of the health services (Donovan 1986). Healthcare beliefs, however, change as younger generations are educated in the same school curricula worldwide.

The factfile approach to culture

One approach which has frequently been deployed in writing about ethnic minorities is the 'factfile' approach, which provides a description of the core beliefs and practices of a given cultural group. The factfile approach offers cultural and religious knowledge as a way of solving professional and institutional difficulties in meeting the needs of ethnic minority patients (Gunaratnam 1997). It argues that in order to improve healthcare, minorities should be re-socialized through health education, while at the same time health and service providers must be equipped with the tools of cultural understanding. Such factfiles have been used by palliative care workers and include detailed information about death, dying and bereavement (e.g. Firth 1993a; Neuberger 2004).

Factfiles range in content from well researched and sensitive material (Henley 1987; Neuberger 1987) to simplistic approaches (Bal and Bal 1995). Populations are typically categorized according to beliefs and practices. For instance, Alix Henley provides a list of the cultural customs of different ethnic groups. This approach is problematic in a number of ways. Ahmad (1996: 195) argues that these factfiles or checklists pathologize culture – minority health problems are seen to arise from their own cultural practices. There is a politics of victim blaming:

> In the guise of cultural understanding one is frequently offered a cata-
> logue of checklists of cultural stereotypes which are regarded as essen-
> tial characteristics of particular racial / cultural types and which signify
> the deviance and the peculiarities of minority cultures to the normality
> of 'British' culture.

Culture becomes reified and seen as something which is static, not as some-thing dynamic and negotiated. Factfile approaches provide, as Gunaratnam (1997) argues, snapshots of cultural and religious practices. This approach neglects the historical factors which influence cultural narratives and mystify the social production of culture. Factfile approaches neglect the power relations which continuously destabilize cultural practices.

Factfiles can stereotype people from a different culture, which leads to expectations about how someone from a certain culture should behave. They may detract from individual subjectivity. They privilege and separate cultural processes from individual and subjective elements. Within a given cultural group there may be much inter-individual variation of what people do in relation to health. People do not always behave in terms of their culture. For instance, non-compliance with medication may be seen to be based on cultural beliefs, whereas it may in fact be an idiosyncratic choice.

In summary, factfile approaches are part of the professional discourse on multiculturalism but at the same time use conceptualizations of cultural and religious practices which are silent about racism and can legitimate discrimination (Gunaratnam 1997). Cultural analysis may divert from the more important issue of demonstrating how racism is a common experience of all non-White people, involving them in social disadvantage resulting in higher rates of illness than White people. Ahmad (1993: 2) argues:

> in this perspective, racialised inequalities in both health and access to healthcare are explained as resulting from cultural differences and deficits. Integration on the part of minority communities and cultural understanding and ethnic sensitivity on the part of the health professional then become the obvious solution. Personal and institutional racism and racial discrimination have no part in this equation.

Is culture at all a useful concept when examining ethnic minority health? It is a very nebulous concept, which is often criticized as being a reification and simplification of perennially shifting experience, forcing a picture of predictability and order onto what is essentially chaotic. However, having said this, it *is* an important variable in the perception, experience and expression of suffering and therefore a useful term. There are very real differences between cultural groups. However people may often see themselves as being part of a wider group than their ethnic group. For example, many south Asians define their core identity as Muslim as opposed to relating to nationhood or being non-White. Also there may be broad cognitive structures which differentiate cultural groups and determine how they respond to their (often disadvantaged) position. People actively draw on elements of their culture to manage life stresses. Culture influences, rather than determines, the way people live. It provides ideas about the appropriate behaviour in a given situation, their response to illness and to medical ideas about treatment.

The problem with culturalist explanations of health and health behaviour

In the health related literature on ethnic minorities, there is a strong tendency for explanations of variations in health status in different ethnic communities to be based on oversimplistic culturalistic explanations. These culturalist explanations account for differences in the healthcare needs of Black and ethnic minority people in terms of cultural variations and ignore social and economic deprivation as being causally related to the development of certain illnesses. For instance, rickets among Asian groups is held to relate to the 'Asian diet' and lack of sunlight. The fact that many Asians live in inner city areas with limited access to park space and limited mobility on account of a real fear of racial discrimination is not taken into account. Socio-economic factors are ignored.

The term socio-economic status (SES) is a broad term referring to economic and social circumstances. It is difficult to measure directly and proxy measures, such as occupation of head of the household, are generally used to indicate different socio-economic groups. The distinction between what is ethnic and what is socio-economic is far from clear in minority groups (Nazroo and Davey-Smith 2001). Although differences in socio-economic status or class may be more important than ethnic or cultural differences in explaining ethnic minority health statuses, both culture and ethnicity are still important. In this respect Smaje (1995: 124–5) argues for the importance of 'more refined approaches to the dynamic interactions between culture, socio-economic status and health experience'.

Similarly Ahmad (1996: 215) calls for more sophisticated understandings of the concept of culture:

> In studying health and illness among minority ethnic communities, the cultural context is of crucial importance. However to be of value, either in explanatory or practical terms, 'culture' needs to be recognised as a context, itself flexible and contested, interacting with, shaping and shaped by other social and structural contexts of people's lives. Cultural norms, themselves contested and changing, represent flexible guidelines within which behaviour is negotiated rather than an independent variable which is solely responsible for determining behaviour. Recognising this will be an important development in moving towards research on health and social care of minority ethnic communities which is of value for both its academic and practical contributions.

What relevance does the above hold in relation to cancer? The terms race and ethnicity have little explanatory value in themselves. Consider the question of breast cancer screening. Is the service being accessed by all racial or ethnic groups? If not, why not? Categories used such as South Asian or Black may be crude and the programme may be accessed well by South Asians generally, but Bangladeshi Muslim women may have poor attendances. To answer this question, the South Asian population could be subdivided into Bangladeshi, Indian and Pakistani. However, when data is required for the development of a new policy, to effect change or evaluate the effectiveness of treatment, there is a need for a much deeper understanding (Bhopal 2001). For example, in order to understand why breast screening is taken up less by some racial/ethnic groups it is important to ask about causality issues, religious views, language of communication, beliefs about prevention and understandings of cancer. The attitudes and behaviours of service providers which might lead to racial discrimination are also crucial to further understanding. The terms 'race' and 'ethnicity' cannot answer these questions and the 'Black box of race' and ethnicity needs to be opened (Bhopal 1997). The terms may be markers or indicators of problems which merit further investigation.

The political economy of health and illness

The literature on health and ethnicity, including that on ethnic differences in cancer, often treats ethnicity as a 'social fact' representing a real and significant dimension of social experience. Field *et al.* (1997: 21) have argued that the intention is to establish interrelationships between these different aspects of social reality in order to explain differences in health status and health outcomes. In this 'paradigm', explanations of ethnic differences in mortality and illness behaviour are largely concerned with 'real differences'. This approach is limited to the analysis of patterns of behaviour and of the broad social factors which shape individual behaviour.

What is ignored in this approach is a consideration of the unequal distribution of power and resources within societies and the conflicts around competing interests. In the political economy approach in anthropology (Singer and Baer 1995), explanatory priority is given to the material conditions mediating differences in health and mortality between different groups. This perspective emerged in the early 1980s and adopts a holistic understanding of the causes of sickness. It focuses on the interrelationship of medical systems with political structures, the contested character of provider/patient relations, and locates the patient's/sufferer's experience in political and economic contexts. Beyond underscoring the consequences of power and resources for health and mortality, this approach examines the ways in which power is maintained through the actions and ideas of social groups, such as doctors. In the biomedical approach, with its emphasis upon individuals as the site of disease and upon medical intervention, attention is deflected away from the fundamental underlying social and economic inequalities which are a significant cause of health inequality. A full understanding of health inequalities necessitates an appreciation of these power structure differentials.

Lay theories of health and illness

How a person explains a disease is likely to influence how they respond to it and what they do about it. In many parts of the world where people lack biomedical knowledge, disease is explained in terms of lay theories. There have been several attempts to classify lay illness aetiologies, especially in non-Western societies. For instance, Foster and Anderson (1978) differentiate between personalistic and naturalistic systems. In the former, illness is due to the purposeful active intervention of an agent, such as a God or a ghost. In naturalistic systems, illness is explained in impersonal, systemic terms due to natural forces or conditions, such as cold, wind or damp or disequilibrium within the individual. Helman (2001) describes how lay theories can be divided up into aetiologies in different domains. These domains may vary in emphasis between different cultural groups. Sickness may be 'caused' by various disturbances in:

1 The individual, e.g. genetics, smoking, diet;
2 The natural world, e.g. heat, wind, lunar influence, toxins, viruses;
3 The social world, e.g. witchcraft, sorcery, evil eye;
4 The supernatural world, e.g. gods, spirits.

In most cases lay theories of illness aetiology are multi-causal. Kleinman (1980) describes a framework for eliciting patient's 'explanatory models' about specific diseases. Explanatory models are sets of beliefs or understandings that specify how an illness episode is caused, its mode of onset and symptoms, pathophysiology and its treatment. These are formed and employed to cope with specific health problems and therefore need to be analysed in that concrete setting (Dein 2004a).

Explanatory models are attributes of individuals. They draw on shared cultural knowledge but remain at least partially idiosyncratic and situational. They are frequently fragmented, not fully worked out and often change and are influenced by the individual's illness experiences and treatments. They are related to help-seeking behaviour in complex ways. They provide patients with the information they need when choosing and evaluating medical interventions, communicating with others about sickness and making their own distress recognizable to them. Being pragmatic they are strongly orientated to making statements about illness causation. Patients and physicians may hold different explanatory models of illness deriving from their differential knowledge of medicine and this fact might result in problems in doctor-patient communication and interaction. These explanatory models may relate in specific types of health seeking behaviour and should be elicited from patients and their families so that physicians can understand specific illness behaviours.

Beliefs about cancer may influence the perception of risk of developing the disease, participation in screening programmes, emotional responses to the disease, doctor-patient relationships and decisions about treatments, and are therefore of importance to oncologists and other health professionals working with cancer patients (Cooley and Jennings-Dozier 1998). It is important to differentiate lack of biomedical knowledge from lay beliefs. A person may have little understanding of the factors causing cancer, or on the other hand, may hold lay beliefs which differ significantly from biomedical understandings.

Western societies predominantly stress factors within the individual or natural world, whereas explanations involving the social world or supernatural worlds are still commonplace in traditional societies, where religious worldviews prevail. For instance, in one study, Latina women in southern California were more likely to attribute breast cancer to 'sinful' behaviour (alcohol and drug use) than Anglo-American women (Chavez et al. 1995). It appears that modernization and globalization might be eroding these traditional belief systems, although indigenous people may still maintain them to a greater or lesser degree (see Box 1.1).

Explanatory models can have practical implications. In some instances holding idiosyncratic beliefs about cancer may inhibit the use of biomedical treatments. A study of disadvantaged Hispanic women in the Bronx, New York, found that 58 per cent believed that surgical treatment of breast cancer would cause it to metastasize. Holding such beliefs might prevent women from undergoing potentially curative treatments such as lumpectomy (Morgan *et al.* 1995).

Eliciting explanatory models about cancer

Lay beliefs about cancer may be elicited in four major ways:

1 Structured interviews using rating scales;
2 Ethnographic interviews;

Box 1.1 Explanatory models of sickness among the Navaho

Among the American Navaho Indians, serious illness such as cancer is attributed to a number of causes including: soul loss; intrusive objects; spirit intrusion or possession; breach of taboo or witchcraft/sorcery. Religion permeates all aspects of life (Kittler and Sucher 1998). Healing is considered sacred work and is not considered effective without considering the spiritual aspect of the individual. Use is made of traditional healing and biomedicine simultaneously.

In one study (Diversity Resources Inc. 2001) 70 per cent of Navahos used traditional healers and 28 per cent of Indians living in Milwaukee and the San Francisco Bay area continued to use traditional healers. It is seen as acceptable for a person to consult a Navaho diagnostician to identify the *cause* of a disease and arrange a ceremony to eliminate that cause, as well as to consult a physician to alleviate the *symptoms* of the disease. Traditional healers may burn herbs in an abalone shell to purify people and places in a ceremony called *smudging*. Sickness of any degree is seen to affect the whole community and healing is a communal affair. In traditional Navaho medicine, illnesses are classified by the agents believed to cause them or the ceremonies used to cure them rather than by parts of the body affected. Cancer may not be discussed publicly to avoid 'wishing' it on others (Glanz 2003).

3 Semistructured interviews;
4 Focus groups.

A number of quantitative scales have been devised to measure beliefs about cancer including the Black American (American Cancer Society 1981), adolescent perception (Price *et al.* 1998) and the Chinese Beliefs Questionnaire (Dodd *et al.* 1985) based on Kleinman's idea of explanatory models. These scales measure attitudes towards and beliefs about cancer, cancer prevention and cancer treatments within a variety of age groups and ethnic populations. They vary in their validity and reliability (Nielson *et al.* 1992). They are generally quick and easy to administer and can be analysed using routine statistics. However, like most structured questionnaire studies, they impose definitions on informants (such as perceived causes of cancer) without allowing for the informants own (or emic) definitions of what is going on. A good example of the use of quantitative methodology is a study which examined the psychosocial factors influencing attendance, non-attendance and re-attendance in a breast screening programme in an inner city area in the UK (Fallowfield *et al.* 1990). This study deployed quantitative rating scales, devised by the researchers who examined health beliefs, knowledge about cancer and attitudes towards breast cancer screening.

In ethnographic interviews the researcher elicits an in-depth account of how informants themselves understand a particular disease 'the essential principle in developing an understanding of a person's beliefs is to try and understand the world . . . through that person's eyes' (Sensky 1996: 64). The interviewer does not pursue any a priori assumptions and attempts to move outside any ethnocentric views. Unlike quantitative studies, qualitative interviews are carried out on small numbers of informants to obtain in-depth information. They are analysed by content analysis, whereby themes are drawn out from the data. Data from qualitative interviews can be used to devise quantitative scales.

Semistructured interviews can be used to elicit informants' models of illness. Here the interviewer asks about a range of topics which informants can elaborate upon. A study by Gifford (1994) examining 20 middle-aged working-class women of Italian Australian descent, looked at understandings of cancer using in-depth semistructured interviews. This study is illustrative of studies in the literature which deploy qualitative methods and demonstrates the different meanings one group holds about cancer. Cancer was attributed by informants to the menopause where blood no longer flowed and therefore became putrid leading to cancer. The word cancer was used reluctantly by these women. Instead they used the euphemism 'that terrible disease'. Included in the rubric cancer were a number of tumours both benign and malignant. Only malignant tumours were held to be fatal. By contrast benign tumours were cancers that could be cured and were described as being 'little, centred in one place, not having roots and not being in the blood'. Malignant tumours were held to have roots and spread through the blood. On account of this, cutting out the tumour could not be successful. The perceived prognosis for this malignant tumour was almost inevitably death.

Several women held that if a doctor discovered a malignant tumour, the woman should not be told for fear that death could be hastened. A third group of conditions were not considered to be tumours but could turn into tumours if not treated. This group included fibroids, cold sores, inflammation and cysts. Generally cancer was held to be asymptomatic and was frequently discovered too late when the roots had spread. Other proposed causes of cancer were sorrow, unhappiness and living an unnatural life.

Another qualitative method is the use of focus groups. Here a group of 6–12 participants are interviewed together. Use is made of the group dynamic to focus on a particular topic, for instance health beliefs. Participants may be asked to discuss various audiovisual media, such as leaflets or videos. Dein (2005) has deployed this methodology to understand attitudes towards cancer among elderly Bangladeshis in London (see Box 1.2). In this study informants held cancer to be incurable and a disease that doctors could not do much about. It is not surprising that this population is reluctant to seek help for cancer.

Bangladeshis aside, there has been little work examining knowledge and understandings of cancer in the UK among other ethnic minority groups (Dein 2004a). In one study of cancer beliefs among the White majority

---

Box 1.2 Attitudes of elderly Bangladeshis to cancer: focus group study

Cancer is invariably fatal.

'If you have it you will die, that's certain. It's always fatal' (male, 65 years)

There is nothing that doctors can do about cancer.

'I don't think any treatment helps cancer. Once you have it, there is nothing you can do. It will kill you.' (male, 60 years)

Cancer is a horrible death.

'I knew of one man who had cancer in Bangladesh. He went yellow and lost weight. He had a lot of pain and died soon after. It was a horrible death.' (male, 56 years)

Doctors are not good at picking up cancer.

'Doctors do not treat us well, they do not respect us. They do not examine people properly and I don't think they can pick up cancer.' (woman, 51 years)

community in the UK, the perceived causes ranged from moral wrongdoing to contagion (Box 1984). Other perceived causes include trauma caused by divorce or separation (Bhopal and Rankin 1996). In Baxter's (1989) study, there was a clear lack of knowledge about cancer especially among non-English speaking and older people. Of interest, the beliefs of the minority groups did not differ widely from those of the majority White population. Cultural beliefs related to sexuality may influence treatment decisions. West Indian women in the UK are reluctant to have a hysterectomy, since they consider that menstruation is a cleansing act clearing the body of impurity. Following surgery they see themselves as less of a woman and are afraid that their partner may go off them (Rider 1997). In another study it was found that those considering themselves to be healthy and fit (and therefore not harbouring any serious disease) did not understand the concept of screening (Hoare 1996).

The relevance of cultural epidemiology

Although the health beliefs in a population are likely to relate in some way to what people actually do in practice, it is essential to have a knowledge of how these beliefs are distributed in a population. Much of the health belief literature is predicated upon the rather naïve idea that if health beliefs can be elicited from a small sample of the population (qualitative studies typically deploy 20–40 participants or so) these beliefs will apply to the whole population. This is based upon a simplistic notion of culture as being homogenous and health beliefs being part of that culture. It is important to see how these beliefs are distributed within a population using epidemiological techniques. Only by doing this can health interventions be planned and implemented. It is not enough to use small scale qualitative studies to plan health interventions; these studies provide the basis for further quantitative studies. Both qualitative and quantitative studies are essential for health education and intervention programmes. For a good discussion of this approach in psychiatry and tropical medicine see Weiss (2001).

The metaphorization of cancer

Anthropologists describe how disease labels can be applied to society and similarly social labels (usually pejorative) are often applied to certain diseases. Cancer has occasioned a constellation of metaphorical systems. Even the name cancer itself is a metaphor deriving from the Latin word for crab denoting a swollen protuberance like the legs of a crab. In contemporary Western society cancer is fraught with fantasies of rot invading the body and animals that gnaw and destroy it (Herzlich and Pierret 1987: 56).

In the UK a number of metaphors are used for cancer relating to its severity and evasion of medical treatments. These include 'unrestrained', 'uncontrollable', 'chaotic' or 'evil force' – a disease which might afflict any-one at any time in any place. In the popular imagination cancer equals death (Sontag 1989). It is a disease which in modern Western societies is often viewed as being brought upon oneself through irresponsibility, bad diet, smoking or by the suppression of angry or negative thoughts (Lupton 2004).

The metaphors carry a range of symbolic associations and determine to some extent how sufferers perceive their own condition and how other people respond to them. Metaphors may be stigmatizing and might lead to avoidance of those with the condition. Peters-Golden (1982) has described how the stigma associated with breast cancer can result in other people avoiding the sick person possibly on account of the belief that the disease is in some way contagious. One study in Italy indicated that women them-selves may see breast cancer as a 'plague', a malevolent force that has invaded them from the outside (Gordon and Paci 1997).

The dominant discourse surrounding cancer in modern society today is that of 'hope'. This postulates that winning the 'war' against cancer is intim-ately linked to having a positive attitude to getting better. This discourse emphasizes 'will' and the idea that 'if one has enough hope, one may will a change in the course of the disease in the body' (Good *et al.* 1990: 62) hence underlining notions of individualism, fighting spirit and the power of thought in contemporary American society. These beliefs can lead to demoralization, depression and self blame when the cancer patient fails to be cured or the cancer returns. This discourse supports the current ethic of disclosure in the USA.

The militarization metaphor of 'fighting' is also prevalent. Erwin (1987) argues that the militarization metaphor for cancer leads to the expectation that patients will 'fight' the cancer. Cowardice, giving in, fear and denial are not considered socially acceptable ways of dealing with the disease. Opti-mism and positive coping are expected. Similar attitudes relate to physicians treating the cancer (Erwin 1987: 21): 'For the medical doctor the long range goal is to determine which treatment protocols produce the best statistical curves – that is, in his opinion, the way to win the war. The war is his career. Fighting a single battle is the concern of the individual patient/soldier'.

Concepts of the self, autonomy, agency and responsibility

Cultural conceptualizations relating to the self and autonomy may be cross-culturally variable and this may have significant implications for the treat-ment of cancer in these groups. It cannot be assumed that the dualisms we take for granted in Western culture occur worldwide. Self–other and mind/body dualisms may be specifically Western cultural constructs. Notions of the person and self vary across the world. One broad generalization is that in non-Western cultures notions of self and personhood are closely tied to belonging to a social group. The notion of the unique, bounded, rational, autonomous individual is a Western construct (see Morris 1994; Markus and Kitayama 1991 for a good discussion of cultural aspects of the self).

For instance, in Africa, Nobels (1991: 55) points out how:

> Unlike Western philosophical systems, the African philosophical tradition does not place heavy emphasis on the individual – whatever happened to the individual happened to the corporate group, the tribe, and whatever happened to the tribe happened to the individual ... a cardinal point to understand the traditional African's view of himself, his self concept, is that he believes 'I am, because we are; and because we are, therefore I am'.

In African American communities unity and kinship are valued. Self-preservation and individualism are not valued. This is significant in the planning and implementation of community based health programmes. Failure to include community members in cancer screening programmes' design and their implementation and evaluation, interrupts collective unity and kinship (Jennings 1996).

There may be significant cross-cultural differences in the ways that individuals are held accountable for their illnesses. Especially in the Western world, ill health is increasingly blamed on not taking care of one's diet, dress, hygiene, lifestyle, relationships, sexual behaviour, smoking and drinking habits and physical exercise. The extent to which people believe their health is determined by their own actions as opposed to luck, chance or external factors correlates with socio-economic variables (Pill and Stott 1982). The term 'agency' refers to intention or consciousness of action, sometimes with the implication of possible choices between different actions. The sense of personal control may be culturally variable. In India, for instance, patients' feeling of well-being depends less on a sense of personal control than in the West (Saxena 1994). The family plays a significant role at each stage of diagnosis and management (Chaturvedi 1994). There is a similar state of affairs among certain ethnic minorities in the USA (Meyerowitz *et al.* 1998).

In Britain and the USA sick patients and their families make use of an explanatory framework which often includes a moral or quasi-moral judgement. The individual is held accountable for various disorders to different degrees. Diabetes, along with some cancers, brain haemorrhages and many common infectious diseases stand at the least blame end of the spectrum. The individual is generally not held to be responsible for developing these disorders. Sexually transmitted diseases, cirrhosis of the liver and lung cancer are more strongly associated with a personal contribution towards the cause of the suffering (Crawford 1980). The allocation of 'blame' to individual sufferers of illness to some extent will determine their responses to this illness.

Locus of control and fatalism

Culture determines how people respond to misfortune. In groups who hold a fatalistic outlook on life, the belief may be held that the individual cannot necessarily exercise control over his or her health. This attitude, which sees health as being largely determined by forces outside the control of the individual and thus denies the relevance of individual behavioural change, is referred to as fatalism. As will be discussed below, fatalistic attitudes towards cancer are still prevalent in many parts of the world. Davison *et al.* (1992) point out how the Western approach to health education takes individual control as correct, whereas belief in other agencies requires rectification (usually education). Health promotion is seen as a struggle between a modern belief in lifestyle and an outdated belief in fatalism. However attempts to modify lifestyle to prevent disease onset in groups who hold fatalistic outlooks on life may not be well received. In such groups holding fatalistic ideologies, patients with cancer may 'accept' their imminent demise and refuse potentially life-saving treatment. Psychosocial responses including fear, underestimation, fatalism and pessimism have been identified as factors inhibiting Black American patients from participating in health promotion behaviour (Jennings 1996; Long 1993). Cultural groups differ significantly in the degree to which fatalism is part of their general worldview.

Narrative in medical anthropology

The study of language has close ties to the study of culture. This relationship was perhaps best illustrated by Claude Levi-Strauss's work on structuralism (Levi-Strauss 1958) which applied linguistic theories to 'explain' cultural phenomena. In the past decade all areas of the humanities and social sciences have developed an increasing preoccupation with language, and an increasing recognition and understanding of the role of language in constituting and maintaining notions of reality. This reflects the 'linguistic turn' in the philosophy of science' (Kvale 1992), characterized by a change in emphasis from a confrontation with nature to a focus on conversation, and from a correspondence with an objective reality to the negotiation of meaning. There has been a shift from psyche to text. Language is seen as possessing the power to create and organize our experiences.

Related to this is the contemporary emphasis on the pervasiveness of stories in all human thought and action (Dein 2004b). Over the last decade, narrative has been a subject of increasing interest among social scientists. The term 'narrative' relates to the telling of some true or fictitious event, or connected sequence of events, in which the events are selected and arranged in a particular order (the plot). According to the narrative approach, we live in a 'storied' world, we make sense of things by telling stories to ourselves and others.

A number of social scientists have focused on narrative specifically within the realm of illness. Recording and analysing the narratives of patients and professionals can provide key insights into beliefs, attitudes, behaviours and barriers to change. Kleinman (1990) in his *The Illness Narratives: Suffering, Healing and the Human Condition* argues that doctors need to listen to the patient's story about their illness in order to understand their illness experience. Good (1994: 133) posits that narrativization is a process through which the lifeworld of the sick patient, shattered by illness, is reconstituted. Similarly Skultans (1998: 232) argues for narrative resulting in a reconstruction of the self and identity for the sick person:

> Everyday routines and relationships, hitherto taken for granted, are disrupted, and explanations can no longer be met. Sometimes these changes require a fundamental reconstruction of one's sense of self and identity. Narrative is the means by which such changes can be brought about, since personally constructed stories about the self provide a space in which values can be reasserted and new roles described.

It is perhaps Frank (1997), a sociologist and himself a sufferer from cancer, in his book *The Wounded Story Teller: Body, Illness and Ethics*, who most persuasively writes about the principal plots of Western illness narratives: the restitution, the chaos, the quest and the testimonial narrative. He points out that in any illness, all four narrative types are told alternatively and repeatedly. Each narrative reflects strong cultural and personal preferences and is shaped by existing genres of storytelling in a society. The restitution narrative dominates stories of most people who have become recently ill and sometimes those who are chronically ill. By restitution he means narratives characterized by 'yesterday I was healthy, today I'm sick, but tomorrow I'll be healthy again'. However bad things look, a happy ending is possible. Clinicians cannot entertain the chaos narrative (its plot imagines life never getting better) since it threatens the 'triumph of modernity' including the power of biomedicine. Frank writes (1997: 112) 'The restitution narrative demands hegemony: it denies chaos and requires chaotic bodies to be depressed and thus fixable'.

Cancer destroys the 'taken for grantedness' of everyday life and results in fear and uncertainty. It results in 'suffering', a term commonly deployed by those with the illness and one that is difficult to define. Cassell (1982: 639) refers to suffering as relating to a number of interconnected threats and losses: losses to personhood; threats to the identity; threats to the person's future; threats to self-image; a perceived lack of options for coping; a sense of personal loss and a lack of a basis for hope. He goes on to state how

> the test of medicine should be its adequacy in the face of suffering . . . modern medicine fails that test. In fact the central assumptions on which twentieth Century medicine is founded provide no basis for an understanding of suffering. For pain, difficulty in breathing, or other difficulties of the body, superbly yes, for suffering no.
>
> (Cassell 1982: 639)

In a similar way the Irish palliative care physician Michael Kearney (1997) states how the medical model is aptly able to deal with the physical aspects of pain but is unable to deal with the nature of suffering entailing threatened loss to the integrity of the person.

This loss of a sense of bodily integrity is well illustrated in a study by Chattoo *et al.* (2002) which used in-depth qualitative interviews to elicit the narratives of South Asian (Indian, Pakistani and Bangladeshi origin) and White people with advanced cancer and their carers in the UK. They used a biographical approach and compared narratives across families and ethnic groups to understand the salience of ethnicity in relation to gender, age and socio-economic position in shaping the illness and caring experience of the research participants. This study illustrates the centrality of the notion of discontinuity and fractured self in understanding the impact of cancer on different aspects of identity and points to the difficulty in the re-negotiation of identity in relatively young communities where the experience of cancer is far less common than in the White population.

There is a growing awareness of the role that narratives play in helping cancer patients cope with their illness. Narratives can be deployed to objectify and distance oneself from problems, to gain understanding, establish meaning, develop greater self knowledge and decrease emotional distress. In relation to this, Carlick and Biley (2004) argue that there is a need for health professionals to incorporate the use of narratives into their practices. To date, however, the cross-cultural study of cancer narratives is in the embryonic stage. In terms of cancer, cultures may differ in the ways that they recount their 'cancer narratives'. These may have significant implications for communication and treatment. Although little studied, this is a fruitful area for further research. Potential areas might include the ways that different groups structure their narratives and the influence of 'cultural narratives' on individual response to cancer and its healing. Beyond this there is some anecdotal 'evidence' that the recitation of narratives might themselves be 'healing' for cancer patients.

The expression of emotion

Cultural factors determine the ways in which symptoms are expressed and the psychological response to cancer. Although far from simple, anthropological experience in non-Western cultures suggests that the Cartesian split between mind and body which we find in Western cultures is not present in other parts of the world. In Western society the duality of mind and body is hierarchical, with intellect over emotions and the soma. Somatic distress is seen as secondary communication of primary psychological distress. In contrast, in other cultures, such as Buddhist and Hindu traditions, feelings and intuitions have a higher value than words and the emotional response to cancer may be predominantly somatic – that is expressed through bodily symptoms. Somatic presentation of complaints is not related to a lack of vocabulary or sophistication of psychological processing as much as to a conceptual difference in the primacy of the body as the appropriate vehicle of communication for both physical and emotional distress (Kagawa-Singer *et al.* 1997).

Somatization, the expression of psychological distress through physical symptoms, is common in non-European cultures (Jablensky *et al.* 1981; Marsella *et al.* 1985; Ramirez *et al.* 1991). The phenomenon of somatization may be frequently found in certain ethnic minority populations in the West including Indians, Pakistanis and Bangladeshis (Bal 1987; Mumford 1993). Some cultures may have difficulty using the word depression. For instance, Muslims may not use the word depression since feeling depressed demonstrates a lack of respect for Allah.

Understanding these idioms of distress has important implications for health professionals working with cancer patients. Failure to understand the mode of emotional expression might result in an overemphasis on physical symptoms and the neglect of underlying psychological distress.

Summary

The above discussion illustrates the variety of ways in which cultural factors may influence understandings of and attitudes towards cancer and the response to it. A problem for medical anthropologists is how to incorporate these anthropological themes into practice and to develop a clinically applied anthropology. This is discussed in following chapters. These themes will recur throughout the book and have significant implications for those working with cancer patients from various cultural groups. In particular, the book will adopt a critical stance towards concepts such as culture and ethnicity. Working with ethnic minority groups involves more than just addressing the 'problem of culture'; it must extend to an examination of the wider social constraints – including racism and discrimination – in which these cultural beliefs are embedded.

Further reading

Brown, P.J. (1998) *Understanding and Applying Medical Anthropology*. Mountain View, CA: Mayfield.

Hahn, R. (1995) *Sickness and Healing: An Anthropological Perspective*. New Haven: Yale University Press.

Helman, C. (2001) *Culture, Health and Illness*. London: Hodder Arnold.

Johnson, T. and Sargent, C. (1996) *Medical Anthropology: Contemporary Theory and Method*. Westport, CT: Praeger.

Keesing, R. and Strathern, N. (1997) *Cultural Anthropology: A Contemporary Perspective*. Forth Worth: Harcourt Brace.

Pelto, P. and Pelto, G. (1978) *Anthropological Research: The Structure of Inquiry*. Cambridge: Cambridge University Press.

2 Screening and cancer prevention across cultures: moving beyond culture

The role of individual medical care in preventing sickness and premature death is secondary to that of other influences, yet society's investment in healthcare is based on the premise that it is the major determinant. It is assumed we are ill and made well, but it is nearer the truth that we are well and made ill.

(McKeown 1979)

There is evidence that certain measures may be effective in preventing the onset of cancer. These range from lifestyle changes relating to exercise, occupation, smoking, alcohol and diet to formal cancer screening which can pick up early or premalignant disease. This chapter examines the influence of cultural factors on preventive behaviour including screening. It focuses on studies in the USA/Canada, Australia and the UK. After discussing the concept of prevention and the types of prevention, the influence of cultural beliefs on screening programmes will be examined, emphasizing the problems regarding the notion of 'cancer fatalism'. Finally, recent work on ethnicity and genetic screening will be outlined.

How meaningful is the concept of prevention?

To date there has been little anthropological work examining how different cultural groups understand the notion of prevention. To prevent illness means planning ahead. This may be an alien concept in communities that are affected by hunger and poverty, where life is unpredictable and precarious and people may 'live for the moment'. To talk to poverty stricken communities about eliminating risk factors such as smoking to prevent the development of lung cancer twenty years later, not only does not make sense to them, it is simply impractical. It has been argued that this concept of health prevention is based on a 'middle class investment model' which emphasizes investment now to 'reap' a healthy future. This value cannot be easily applied to all groups of people (Helman 2001).

Types of prevention

Cancer prevention can occur at three levels: primary, secondary and tertiary. Primary prevention refers to preventing or eliminating exposure to carcinogenic substances with the aim of preventing the cancer process from occurring. Non-smoking, avoiding sunburn or avoiding exposure to ionizing radiation are good examples. Other examples include preventing the spread of viruses such as HIV, which increase the risk of developing certain types of cancer. For primary prevention the cause of the cancer must be known.

Secondary prevention, or screening, refers to detecting the cancer early to improve the chances of successful treatment. Examples include the Pap test for cervical cancer, breast self-examination and mammography for breast cancer, digital rectal examination for prostate cancer and testicular self-examination for testicular cancer.

Tertiary prevention refers to the treatment of cancer patients to prevent premature death and to maximize the quality of life for these patients. This will form the subject matter of Chapter 5.

Perceptions of what constitutes a risk factor may differ between the lay public and health professionals and may vary across cultural groups. For instance, a study of beliefs about cervical cancer showed a significant difference between the beliefs of Latina immigrants, who viewed cervical cancer as a moral problem, the consequence of 'immorality' and 'promiscuity' and therefore highly stigmatized, and those of their physicians who saw it as a preventable disease (Chavez *et al.* 1995; Chavez *et al.* 1999). The Latina immigrants often considered cancer to be caused by sugar substitutes, bruises, microwave ovens, eating pork, breastfeeding and antibiotics (Perez Stable *et al.* 1992). These are not generally considered risk factors by biomedical practitioners.

Lack of biomedical knowledge about a disease can result in lay theories. In a qualitative study of 50 South Asian women (30–72 years) in Western Canada, subjects proposed five domains of belief relating to the development of breast cancer: damage to the breast; contagion; bringing it upon oneself through negative lifestyle; the hands of others (careless words, curses, divine power); and lastly passed down in the family (Johnson *et al.* 1999). Again, apart from genetic factors, the first four domains are not generally considered by biomedical practitioners to be risk factors for breast cancer. In fact, the belief that breast cancer could be contagious might increase the stigma associated with this disease.

Members of a group may share a common explanatory model of their illnesses, something that anthropologists refer to as a 'folk model of illness'. However, not every member of an ethnic group holds identical beliefs about health and illness. Healthcare professionals, therefore, need to understand the range of health beliefs in a population and be sensitive to the possibility that cultural factors may interfere with effective communication (Hahn 1999).

'Culture' in epidemiological studies of risk factors for cancer

Recently epidemiologists of cancer have incorporated culture and ethnicity into their studies. While this is to be applauded, there are problems with the use of the term 'culture' in these contexts. Only 'others' (defined in class, ethnic, or behavioural terms) have culture. The term is rarely used in relation to indigenous White people. Culture may be understood either as a 'protective' factor or as a 'risk' factor, but mainly it is a 'risk' factor. This case is explicitly argued in an article comparing 'Anglo' to 'Latino' perceptions about cancer in the USA (Perez-Stable *et al.* 1992). The Latino high fibre diet and lower smoking rates for women are associated with lower cancer death rates than for the US population as a whole. However, what starts as a 'protective' factor quickly becomes a 'risk' factor: Latinos are held to be under-educated and fatalistic. 'Latino fatalism' then develops into a 'disease' requiring culturally specific 'treatment' to maintain a lower cancer death rate. Instead of concluding that Latinos might be doing the right thing, the authors conclude that because Latinos have a 'culture' they must be doing something wrong.

How does culture influence the perception of risk?

There is to date a limited literature on the ways in which cultural factors influence the perception of risk of developing specific diseases. Weinstein (1987) uses the term 'optimistic bias' to refer to the tendency to view oneself as invulnerable (or less likely than others) to experiencing negative life events. Optimistic bias is a robust finding which has been replicated in a number of contexts including HIV / AIDS, STD and smoking risk and cancer.

In American culture the media permeates every aspect of life emphasizing the idea that the individual is responsible for his or her own health. For this reason Americans may have greater sensitivity to health relevant information and a heightened awareness of their vulnerability to illness compared to other groups. For instance, Fountaine and Smith (1995) found that Americans were more realistic about their chances of developing cancer than the British. The authors speculated that the higher optimistic bias among the British may be due to a lower prevalence of health sensitivity on account of the media exposure in American culture. This assertion is difficult to prove empirically, but may warrant further consideration. There is clearly a need for further research to specifically examine how different cultural groups understand the concept of risk and how these risks are assessed.

Ethnicity and specific risk factors for cancer: complex relationships

There is growing awareness that cancer prevention needs to take account of potentially modifiable risk factors such as smoking, excessive alcohol consumption, lack of physical activity, nutrition, diet and obesity. The prevalence of these risk factors varies by racial/ethnic group and may influence cancer rates (McGinnis and Foege 1993; Colditz and Gortmaker 1995). Specific ethnic groups may have culture-specific risk factors for cancer, which might relate to use of certain carcinogens such as smoking, diet (for instance the habit of consuming fried meats containing heterocyclic amines) or certain behaviours such as unprotected sexual intercourse. By contrast, certain ethnic groups may actually be *protected* from cancer on account of their diet. For example, Japanese people may be protected from lung cancer through their ingestion of tea which contains antioxidants (Weisburger and Chung 2002). There may be interactions between diet and smoking. Individuals on a protective diet rich in antioxidants may be protected against certain cancers (lung, pancreas, kidney) even if they do smoke. The available epidemiological studies do not generally differentiate accumulative lifetime exposure to behavioural risks from current behaviours as influences on cancer.

Inter-relations between ethnicity, gender and risk factors are often complex. For pancreatic cancer, smoking and obesity related diabetes mellitus are more potent risk factors in African American males than among White males in the USA. For women, obesity and a significant intake of alcoholic drinks play a more important role in the development of this cancer in African American women than among non-Hispanic White women (Ghafoor *et al.* 2002).

In the USA Hispanics and African Americans have higher rates of lung cancer compared to their White counterparts even though, for economic reasons, individuals tend to smoke less. One explanation derives from the fact that many African Americans and Hispanics smoke cigarettes almost up to the filter so that more harmful substances are inhaled. Knowledge of these ethnic-specific risk factors provides opportunities for eliminating them and hence the opportunity for primary prevention.

Although it is recognized that different populations have differential exposure to cancer risk factors, there is some evidence that ethnic and racial groups may differ in their genetic susceptibility to various risk factors. There may be variations in the genes which modulate the impact of environmental carcinogens, for instance by their effects on carcinogen-metabolizing enzymes or on their ability to repair DNA lesions induced by carcinogens. This topic, although of significant interest, will not further be examined here. For a good discussion of this area see Parkin (2001).

There is some evidence that exposure to specific risk factors varies between different cultural groups. This issue will now be discussed, starting with obesity. Rather than giving a comprehensive overview of this area, specific examples will be presented.

Obesity

Inadequate physical activity contributes to obesity and may increase the risk of certain cancers (larynx, lymphoma, small intestine and breast cancer). In breast cancer for example, there is increasing evidence that adult weight gain and central body fat acquisition during the menopause is associated with increased risks of postmenopausal breast cancer (Ballard-Barbush *et al.* 1999). Rates of obesity have soared throughout the world since the mid-1980s as individuals have become more sedentary and have consumed greater amounts of high calorie foods. The World Health Organisation estimates that half the adults in Europe and in the urban areas of some developing countries are now obese and in the USA an estimated 60 per cent of adults are considered overweight, with a body mass index (BMI) of at least 25.

In the USA African American women and American Indian/Alaskan native men and women have higher rates of obesity than the general population. The prevalence of obesity varies slightly with the level of education in men, but is strongly correlated with the level of education in women. There are also variations in obesity prevalence by income, which are greater among women than among men (IARC 2002; Hill *et al.* 2003).

Diet

Diet is strongly influenced by cultural factors. In a British study (McCormack *et al.* 2004) Muslim women from India and Pakistan were almost twice as likely to develop breast cancer than Gujarati Hindu women. The researchers suggest that the trend may be caused by differences in life-style factors, such as diet and body size, between the two groups of women. Compared to Pakistani and Indian Muslim women, the Gujarati Hindu women in this study were more likely to be vegetarian and therefore have more fibre in their diet from a higher intake of fruit and vegetables.

The association between chewing *paan* (betel nut) and oral cancer is well documented among South Asians in the UK. British Asian immigrants have brought the areca nut from India (some via East Africa), Pakistan, Bangladesh, and other countries in the region and its use is culture-bound. Areca nut is the seed of the fruit of the oriental palm *Areca catechu* and is the basic ingredient of a variety of widely used chewed products.

Characteristically, thin slices of the nut, either natural or processed, may be mixed with a variety of substances including slaked lime (calcium hydroxide) and spices such as cardamom, coconut, and saffron. Most significantly, they may be mixed with tobacco products or wrapped in the leaf of the piper betel plant.

Of particular interest in the UK and perhaps other developed countries, is that the use of areca nut persists and its use is often enhanced following migration to the UK. From the medical point of view, the most important consideration is the relation between areca nut use and the development of mouth cancer (oral squamous cell carcinoma) and its precursors leukoplakia and submucous fibrosis (Thomas and Kearsley 1993).

Smoking

Smoking is a major cancer related health issue. In the USA the prevalence of adult cigarette smoking is now highest among American Indian/Alaskan native women followed by American Indian/Alaskan native men. The prevalence of smoking is however considerably lower among Hispanic/Latino women and Asian women compared with non-Hispanic White women. Socio-economic considerations are of importance in this relationship. Regardless of race or ethnicity, men and women whose income is less than twice the poverty level are more likely to be current smokers than those with higher incomes (US Department of Health and Human Services 1998). In one study of African American women (MacDowell *et al.* 2002), college educated African American women were less likely to smoke over a hundred cigarettes a day than non-college educated African American women. Full understanding of the relation between race/ethnicity thus must take account of education and SES.

In the UK Afro-Caribbean men and women and Pakistani men have smoking levels similar to the UK average. However, recent UK surveys suggest that smoking is much more common in Bangladeshi men than among White, Pakistani or Indian men. Rates of smoking are particularly high in Bangladeshi men aged 50–74 (Health Education Authority 2000). Smoking rates are reportedly low in South Asian women (Pooransinh and Ramaiah 2001).

A recent British qualitative study (Bush *et al*. 2003), using community participatory methods, examined the influences on smoking behaviour in the Bangladeshi and Pakistani communities in the UK to inform the development of effective and culturally acceptable smoking cessation interventions. Four dominant, highly inter-related themes emerged which had an important influence on smoking attitudes and behaviour: gender, age, religion and tradition. Smoking was found to be a widely accepted practice in Pakistani and Bangladeshi men and was associated with socializing, sharing and male identity. Among Asian women, smoking was associated with stigma and shame and was often hidden from family members. Peer pressure was an important influence on smoking behaviour in younger people, who attempted to hide their smoking from elders. There were varied and conflicting interpretations of how acceptable smoking was within the Muslim religion. The study concluded that culturally sensitive smoking cessation interventions for Bangladeshis and Pakistanis are needed.

Sexual practices

There is evidence that viral infections can cause certain forms of cancer and may be transmitted through sexual practices or intravenous drug abuse. For instance, hepatitis B and C are associated with increased rates of hepatocellular carcinoma; HIV with increased rates of Kaposi's sarcoma and non Hodgkin's lymphoma, cervical and anal cancer; and human papilloma virus (HPV) is associated with increased rates of cervical cancer. Higher rates of hepatocellular carcinoma among Hispanics, Latinos and Asian Americans are thought to reflect the higher prevalence of chronic hepatitis B infections among recent immigrants, possibly relating to increased rates of unprotected sex or drug abuse in this group (El Sarag 2002). Differential rates of cervical cancer reflect difference in the prevalence of HPV infection among female Mexican immigrants (Giuliano *et al*. 1999). This data underscores the need to have culturally sensitive and competent sexual health promotion in specific ethnic groups (Ward *et al*. 2004).

Knowledge of cancer risk factors and symptoms in the USA and UK

Knowledge of cancer risk factors and symptoms is essential for the prevention of cancer or its early detection. There is evidence that among the general population, and in ethnic minorities specifically, biomedical knowledge about cancer may be lacking. It cannot be assumed that biomedical knowledge about cancer is commonplace. In one study in the USA among a socio-economically deprived population, one third of subjects were unaware of the link between smoking and lung cancer (Loehrer *et al.* 1991). Similarly, a cross-sectional study of 706 Salvadorean men in California asked for general statements relating to cancer, factors causing cancer, factors modifying the chances of getting cancer, the spread of cancer, who is more likely to get cancer and treatment effectiveness. The study suggested that these men lacked knowledge about the risk factors, symptoms of cancer and early detection methods (Duminda *et al.* 1999).

Ethnic minorities in the UK have been shown to possess relatively poor knowledge concerning the link between cigarette smoking and disease and to be less likely to cite smoking as a health risk than the UK population as a whole. The proportion of Afro-Caribbean men (27 per cent) who say their smoking has 'no effect' on their current health is above the general population rate for the UK (12 per cent) as is that among Bangladeshi men (22 per cent) and Pakistani men (20 per cent) (Health Development Agency 2000).

However, it is important not to overemphasize this 'deficit knowledge' approach that compares respondents' knowledge with the current standard biomedical guidelines. Respondents (non-medically trained interview informants) are generally less knowledgeable than their healthcare providers and therefore may rank known biomedical risk factors low. While this approach may indicate how much or little is known in relation to biomedical standards, it does little to enhance knowledge of how informants themselves organize their beliefs about, and comprehend the risk factors for, specific cancers. Members of a cultural group have definite beliefs about risk factors which may derive from a multitude of sources: popular media, conversations with health practitioners and a set of culturally based health beliefs. Similarly, there may be significant differences across cultures in attitudes towards prevention, and the degree to which views about misfortune are generally fatalistic.

Beliefs about cancer risk factors in the American general population

It is not just ethnic minorities who lack knowledge about cancer. A study in the USA by the American Society of Clinical Oncology and Cancer Research and Prevention Foundation (2004) examined the 'myths' about cancer prevention among the general population. Of interest was the fact that out of 1000 adults weighted for race and ethnicity, 88 per cent of the general population believed that cancer could be prevented by personal action. To reduce cancer risk 56 per cent believed that they should change their diet and 50 per cent said they should stop smoking. Rather alarmingly, 12 per cent of respondents said they could do nothing to prevent cancer. Although people generally knew that they could take steps to prevent cancer, they did not necessarily have the information they needed as to what practical actions they could take. The study demonstrated that there was a significant gap in cancer knowledge in the general population, which was not directly related to race and ethnicity. There were six 'myths' or gaps in perception as to what did and did not matter in terms of cancer prevention:

1 *Exercise will not reduce my risk of cancer.* Only one half of respondents agreed the risk of cancer could be reduced through exercise. This is contrary to scientific data, which suggests that exercise does in fact reduce cancer risk (Brown *et al.* 2003).

2 *What I eat does not matter when it comes to cancer prevention.* Only 38 per cent of respondents held that eating the right amount of fruit and vegetables every day reduced cancer risk. There is, in fact, evidence that a diet high in fruit and vegetables and low in animal fat and calories can reduce the risk of common cancers such as colonic cancer (Flood *et al.* 2002).

3 *Being overweight does not increase my cancer risk.* Only one third of respondents held that maintaining a healthy weight could reduce cancer risk. In fact, maintaining a healthy weight is one of the best ways of reducing the risk of cancer of the colon, pancreas and breast (Harvie 2003).

4 *I only need to apply sunscreen before going to the beach or pool.* Only one third of the respondents said they applied sunscreen before going to the beach or pool. Skin cancer is the commonest preventable cancer in the USA.

5 *If someone in my family has cancer, I'm not at increased risk for the disease.* Thirty-four per cent of the sample agreed that they were at increased risk of cancer if a family member had had cancer. In fact, if a first-degree relative has had cancer, they are at increased risk of cancer themselves. However, only about 5 to 10 per cent of cancers (including breast, ovary and colon) have a hereditary component.

6 *Taking vitamins or herbal supplements will reduce my chance of getting cancer.* Thirty per cent of the sample strongly endorsed this statement. In fact, a study in 1996 showed that people who smoked and took Beta Carotene were more at risk of lung cancer than those who did not take the supplement (Russell 2002).

Even for common cancers, such as breast cancer, the general population may be lacking in knowledge. In one study among the general population in the UK (Grunfield *et al.* 2002), women were found to have limited knowledge of their relative risk of developing breast cancer, of associated risk factors and of the diversity of potential breast cancer related symptoms. These findings are significant and may relate to the fact that there is a delay of 12 weeks or more in approximately 20–30 per cent of women from the discovery of a breast symptom to presentation to a healthcare provider – a delay which might result in a worsened prognosis.

Interventions to influence cancer risk factors

Given the epidemiological evidence suggesting that racial and ethnic differences in behavioural risk factors do explain some of the racial/ethnic differences in cancer, it may be possible to provide interventional programmes aimed at reducing levels of these specific risk factors. There are good examples in the literature of successful intervention studies that reduce cancer risk. For instance, studies of smoking cessation and reduction in lung cancer in young people are fairly conclusive (Peto *et al.* 2000). The prevention of breast, cervical and colorectal cancer through lifestyle changes in the general population is receiving increasing interest and support.

Overall, there is strong evidence from epidemiological studies of the importance of individually modifiable behavioural risks in cancer aetiology and severity, but there is almost no experimental evidence suggesting that altering behaviours actually has an effect on cancer rates or outcomes. Primary healthcare practitioners and other health professionals can be effective in motivating people to engage in such health risk management programmes. There is a need for research which specifically examines ways of engaging and maintaining participation of ethnic minority groups in effective and efficacious physical activity, nutrition/weight management, smoking cessation and multi-component interventions.

As with all behavioural programmes, the problems of motivation and engagement need to be addressed. This requires a tailored and culturally sensitive health risk management programme in order to overcome significant issues of mistrust and barriers to basic access to primary care. This task requires the intervention of a person with a strong connection to the community being served. Such a person requires skills in motivating others, skills in benefit counselling and enrolment and links to primary care practitioners, healthcare systems and community prevention services. Community health workers – or similar paraprofessionals – can fulfil these roles. They offer linguistic skills and can help beneficiaries get coverage, develop more continuous relationships with a useful source of care, understand current risk behaviours, motivate them to engage in risk management and to receive support and encouragement for maintaining these efforts.

Another possible way of motivating some ethnic groups is through religious organizations such as churches. These may run risk education and reduction programmes for their local communities. Pederson *et al.* (2000), in a review of 56 studies of smoking cessation programmes among African Americans, concluded that church-based interventions might be useful in reducing smoking rates in this group, although the evidence for this was equivocable in this study.

Culture and screening

Screening for breast cancer in the USA among ethnic minority groups

Despite the fact that mammography is a valuable tool for detecting early breast cancer, there is evidence that mammography is underused by Black women. This may result in late presentations of disease. Black women often hold negative attitudes and perceptions that involve images of death, feelings of fear and concerns about unrealistic physical impairments that result from breast cancer and therefore may avoid screening (Frisby 2002). Similar results were found in a study deploying focus groups of African American women (Bailey *et al.* 2000). In this study breast cancer was held to be fatal and a White woman's disease with a stigma attached. There was a direct relationship between these cultural beliefs and the under-utilization of mammography.

Factors such as reliance on God to cure cancer, reluctance for a woman to discuss a potential cancer with her husband or male partner, a general fatalism or lack of knowledge that a breast lump can be serious, even if it is not painful, may detract from help seeking for a potential breast abnormality (Lannin *et al.* 2002). In this study women feared that their husbands would leave them if they found out about a cancer diagnosis which might result in them becoming unattractive or a burden on their partners. Another study among African Americans looked at the determinants of participation in cancer screening. The results indicated a prevailing perception that such programmes were useful only for those who already had a diagnosis of breast cancer (Millon-Underwood *et al.* 1993).

Loehrer *et al.*'s (1991) study of 128 African American and White breast cancer patients found different perceptions of cancer among various cultural and social groups. These misconceptions regarding causation and treatment were directly related to increasing age and lack of education. The older and less educated women were more likely to hold the belief that bumps or bruising to the breast caused cancer and that cancer was contagious. African American patients, along with the elderly and less educated White patients, were more likely to accept non-traditional cancer treatments such as salves and vitamins and to hold that surgery could cause the cancer to spread. The authors suggest that these beliefs might inhibit the use of screening and treatment.

Chavez *et al.* (1999) report on an ethnographic study examining beliefs about risk factors for breast cancer among Latinas and Anglo women in Southern California. Using open-ended interviews and a free listing technique (in which informants listed everything that could cause breast cancer and discussed the reasons for this), the authors found that Latinas' level of knowledge and attitudes about breast cancer differed greatly from those of

Anglos and physicians. For example, Latinas believed that physical trauma to the breast and bad behaviours such as illegal drug use were the most important risk factors for breast cancer. Expressions of fatalism were also more common, including the belief that God gave the women breast cancer to punish them for living bad lives. Latina women held that they needed a mammogram *only* if they already had a breast lump.

On the basis of their results the authors planned and evaluated an intervention study based on Bandura's (1977) theory of behavioural change which essentially argues that individuals will change their beliefs about their own abilities once they have experienced mastery of a task. For instance, a woman will be more likely to perform breast self-examination if she feels competent to do so and if a physician validates her findings. The intervention consisted of four stages: improving cancer knowledge; imparting knowledge of breast cancer risk factors; breast self-examination; and information on mammography. Women who participated in this intervention demonstrated improved knowledge about breast cancer and were more proficient in breast self-examination compared to a control group. Those in the intervention group demonstrated small positive changes in the frequency of breast self-examination and obtaining a mammogram.

Case study: breast cancer screening in Asian women in the USA

Asian women in general and Vietnamese women specifically have poor uptakes of breast cancer screening in the USA. Although these women generally have lower rates of breast cancer than the general population, this finding is still worrying considering that continued exposure to environmental factors is likely to cause the incidence rates to increase in this group. The Vietnamese population has been the fastest growing Asian American ethnic group in the United States.

In Vietnam there are a wide range of religions: Taoism, Confucianism, Buddhism, Catholicism, and Indian mysticism. These religions are pervasive and share a common cosmology. Chinese philosophy influences the believer's everyday actions including their healthcare practices. In traditional Chinese medicine illness results from an imbalance of *yin* and *yang* and is seen as a disruption of order and harmony. It is often perceived as a natural occurrence due to improperly stored food or as a result of supernatural forces. It is to be treated with a variety of folk medicines. Taking a lengthy history, physical examination, drawing blood or requiring a patient to undress are seen as signs of incompetence. Traditional healers are expected to diagnose a condition by taking the pulse. Surgery of any kind is seen as a disruption in harmony and should only be carried out as a last resort. Hospitalization often signifies death.

There are two words for breast cancer in the Vietnamese group '*ung thu nhu hoa*' or '*ung thu vu*' in Vietnamese. Pham and McPhee (1992) looking at American Vietnamese women's knowledge, attitudes and practices regarding breast and cervical cancer screening found that over half of their population believed that illnesses were predestined and there was nothing that could be done to prevent cancer. In their study one third of respondents did not know that a breast lump could signify cancer, over half did not know that a family history was a risk factor for breast cancer and 64 per cent had not heard of a mammogram.

However, it was not just cultural beliefs which were a barrier to breast cancer screening. Other factors included lack of a physician's recommendation, the patient's own lack of knowledge, embarrassment, cost and language difficulty. Some women faced with breast symptoms sought the help of traditional healers such as shamans. Traditional beliefs and practices were less significant barriers to healthcare than lack of health insurance and lack of regular healthcare providers. Since Vietnamese women are often unaware of breast screening practices there is a need for clinicians to recommend screening when appropriate (see Little 2001 for a good review of breast cancer in this group).

Cervical cancer in the USA

In relation to cervical cancer, a postal study looking at delays in obtaining cervical screening in a multi-ethnic population (White American, Latinas, Asian Americans) found that delay was more common in Spanish speaking Latinas and women of Asian descent, especially in those who were more fatalistic and endorsed more misconceptions about cancer (Nelson *et al.* 2002). Similar results were found in a study examining the demographic and other predictors of fatalistic beliefs among Hispanic women and Anglo American women in California using both ethnographic interviews and telephone surveys. Latina immigrants (born outside the USA) were more likely than US born Latinas or Anglo American women to hold fatalistic beliefs. Latinas who believed that fate was a risk factor for cervical cancer, that they would rather not know if they had the disease and that there was nothing one could do to prevent it, were significantly less likely than others to report that they had had a Pap smear within the previous three years (Chavez *et al.* 1997).

Cervical cancer is to some extent preventable through screening. Chinese American immigrants are a growing population in the United States. There is evidence that Pap smear testing is less common in Chinese American immigrants than the general population. Using a community based survey (Ralston *et al.* 2003), most cervical cancer risk factors were recognized by less than half of 472 participants in Seattle. This study suggests the need for an increased recognition of cervical cancer risk factors among this group using culturally and linguistically appropriate educational interventions.

Colorectal cancer in the USA

Fatalistic attitudes in some groups have been proposed as causing poorer prognoses in colorectal cancer compared to the majority White population. For example, African Americans have greater colorectal cancer mortality rates compared to the general population, yet are less likely to participate in faecal occult blood testing. This may result from 'cancer fatalism', the belief that death is inevitable when cancer is present (Powe and Johnson 1995).

Screening among ethnic minorities in the UK

Very few studies have measured ethnic differences in the uptake of screening in the UK. Rates of uptake of screening are generally lower in inner city deprived areas compared to the more affluent suburbs (Greater Manchester Breast Screening Service, personal communication). Studies on ethnicity may be confounded by factors such as socio-economic group. When this is accounted for, uptake by Asian women may not necessarily be lower than by other women in the same area, and may be higher for Black than for White women (Hoare 1996).

Luke (1996) points out that there is a need for research examining the uptake of cervical screening among ethnic minority women in the UK and how various groups understand the concept of screening. Uptake has been shown to be lower among Asian women, who may be unaware of the existence and importance of cervical screening services (Doyley 1991).

There have been few interventional studies among ethnic minority women with the explicit aim of increasing screening rates. Kernohan (1996) reports on a pilot study for breast and cervical cancer screening, using a community development approach, involving specially trained health promotion facilitators in Bradford. Participants derived from Asian, Afro-Caribbean, Eastern European and Chinese backgrounds. There were differences in the baseline levels of awareness about cervical and breast cancer across the different ethnic groups. The South Asian women showed the lowest baseline levels of knowledge about breast and cervical cancer and also the most significant improvements. Significant increases in attendance for cervical smear and breast cancer screening were self reported.

McCaffery et al. (2003) conducted a study of attitudes towards HPV testing (HPV is a risk factor for cervical cancer) among White British, Afro-Caribbean, Pakistani and Indian women in the UK. Women were not fully aware of the sexually transmitted nature of cervical cancer and expressed anxiety, confusion and stigma about HPV as a sexually transmitted disease. There were important concerns about the implications of testing positive for their relationships in terms of trust, blame and fidelity and these concerns, although expressed by women from all ethnic groups, were more marked in Indian and Pakistani women, for whom HPV infection (or perceived risk of infection) would have more significant consequences for their families and the wider community. These findings have significant implications for testing for sexually transmitted diseases which could potentially give rise to cancer.

It must be emphasized that non-participation in screening, maintenance of an unhealthy lifestyle and late presentation for professional help may not necessarily result from cultural factors such as fatalism and other health related beliefs. Other factors such as lack of education about symptoms and treatments may be just as important. In the UK anecdotal reports suggest that certain ethnic groups such as Bangladeshi women have low attendance rates for breast and cervical screening. Non-attendance may derive from inaccurate screening registers, poor awareness of minority ethnic groups' naming systems and the return or extended visits of Asian women to the Indian subcontinent. It may be that there is poor comprehension of the concept of screening among ethnic minority women.

However, despite the impression that some ethnic minorities may be reluctant to be screened, a qualitative study in East London looking at women from a number of ethnic groups including Turks, Kurds, Bangladeshis and Chinese speaking women found that generally these women had a positive attitude towards cervical screening, and once they understood the purpose of the test they were enthusiastic about it. Language, administrative issues and concerns about sterility were barriers to screening. The authors suggest that focus groups may improve the numbers attending screening (Naish *et al.* 1994).

Cancer fatalism

Cancer fatalism is a belief that death is inevitable when cancer is present and is often associated with the belief that nothing can be done to help the sufferer. It has frequently been identified as a barrier to participation in cancer screening, detection and treatment. Powe (2003) has provided a comprehensive overview of this area and the discussion below derives from her seminal paper *Cancer Fatalism: The State of the Science*. Until the 2000s, discussions of cancer fatalism were often limited to anecdotal findings and data obtained through the analysis of data from focus groups and interviews. Empirical research seeking to measure cancer fatalism as an independent or dependent variable was sparse. An early study by the American Cancer Society looked at Black American attitudes to cancer and cancer testing (American Cancer Society 1981). This study highlighted many disparities in African Americans and Anglo Americans with regard to knowledge about cancer and health behaviour and found that African Americans underestimated the presence of cancer and were pessimistic about its cure. They were less knowledgeable about cancer compared to Anglo Americans. People with more fatalistic attitudes have been found to be less likely to partake in preventive services (Conrad et al. 1996; Powe 1996).

Since the end of the 1990s there has been a significant increase in research specifically addressing cancer fatalism as an independent or dependent variable. There continues, however, to be a lack of consistency regarding the theoretical or operational definition of fatalism. The current research on cancer fatalism has expanded to encompass its influence at multiple points along the cancer continuum ranging from early detection to treatment to intervention strategies.

Several authors have examined the philosophical and theoretical perspectives underlining cancer fatalism. Freeman (1989) proposed that poverty and fatalism were closely related. According to this perspective, poverty has both a direct and indirect influence on fatalism, influencing factors such as poor education, lack of employment, sub-standard housing, lack of care access and poor healthcare outcomes. Poverty renders the entire worldview fatalistic and engenders an attitude of impotence in the face of illness, just as in every other sphere of life. Given these realities a spiralling, self-fulfilling prophecy effect ensues. For the poor, the focus may be directed towards day-to-day survival as opposed to health promoting or health maintenance activities such as screening, especially when no symptoms are evident. As a result, participation in screening and early detection might not be used as a viable option.

Powe and Johnson (1995) suggest that two distinct factors might converge to influence the experience of fatalism: the universal experiences of 'angst' and 'nihilism'. Angst is defined as a perceived collapse of meaning in the presence of despair about the future. Nihilism is defined as the experience of coping with feelings associated with meaningless, hopelessness and despair. Although these factors are not the cause of fatalism, they are essential in understanding its presence and significance among some African Americans. Both angst and nihilism reflect the prevailing social, political, economic and spiritual ethos among many impoverished ethnic minority groups. Poverty, racism, discrimination, unemployment and inadequate access to care are very much part of their everyday experiences.

Relationships among these forces cannot frequently be separated from the total experience of many African Americans. Hence, cancer fatalism is a situational manifestation in which individuals may feel powerless in the face of cancer. They may view a diagnosis of cancer as a struggle against insurmountable odds. Individuals within families and communities witness 'cycles of cancer diagnosis and death'. Over time, a diagnosis of cancer becomes associated with inevitable death and these experiences and perceptions are reinforced and perpetuated.

However, cancer fatalism is not an all or none phenomenon. Perceptions of cancer fatalism may develop over time, in other words, it may be that at lower levels the perception of cancer fatalism may not adversely affect the cancer screening rate but as the perceptions increase they may exert a negative influence. It is therefore important to understand factors that influence and predict these perceptions and also to determine the point at which perceptions become strong enough to negatively influence cancer screening practices (Powe 2002). This is an empirical question which might constitute the focus of future research.

Perhaps the experience of fatalism is understandable given the life circumstances in which some minority groups live. Straughan and Seow (1998) argue that fatalism should not be seen as irrational. The authors suggest that women who are fatalistic are actually acting rationally when they avoid a screening test, particularly for breast cancer, because their interpretation of the reality is that screening is not beneficial in decreasing the risk of mortality for cancer. They define fatalism as a belief that some health issues are beyond human control on the basis of certain views about luck, fate, predestination and destiny and suggest that 'spirituality' can reduce fatalism by enhancing hope. Perceptions of cancer fatalism and spirituality are not mutually exclusive. Previous research has found that African American women who hold high perceptions of cancer fatalism also have high perceptions of spirituality and that certain components of spirituality can provide a coping strategy to help modify these fatalistic perceptions (Powe 1997).

In summary, the term cancer fatalism has been used in many different ways in the literature. A review of this literature suggests that cancer fatalism is more prevalent among women, older persons, persons with a lower level of education, those with decreased income, and racial and ethnic minority groups. Only one study has addressed the relationship between knowledge of cancer (colorectal) and cancer fatalism (Powe 1995a). This research found that those with lower levels of knowledge of colorectal cancer and screening had high levels of cancer fatalism. Cancer fatalism is believed to play a role in patients' decisions to participate in breast, cervical, colon rectal and skin cancer screening.

It is important to emphasize that cancer fatalism is not the prerogative of ethnic minority groups exclusively and might relate to lower socio-economic status generally. This is illustrated by Balshem's (1993) study among working-class White Americans. She reported how her informants held that to think about cancer and to look for it 'was to tempt fate' and that cancer testing is 'looking for trouble'.

Future research on fatalism

The role of cancer fatalism among patients already diagnosed with cancer has received little attention. Future research should examine the role of cancer fatalism in cancer survivorship, particularly in adherence to treatment regimes and quality of life. It is possible that fatalistic perceptions are manifested differently in patients receiving treatment to those who are not. There is a need to address the role of cancer fatalism among healthcare providers. If patients perceive negative attitudes about screening from their providers the patients may be less likely to follow these recommendations. Overall there is a need for future research to explore the intricacies and inter-relationships between perceptions of cancer fatalism and other barriers to screening.

Interventions to influence cancer fatalism

Only one study among African Americans specifically sought to decrease perceptions of cancer fatalism through an intervention in patients with colorectal cancer. Powe and Weinrich (1999) evaluated a study deploying a 20 minute video entitled 'Telling the Story. To Live is Gods Will'. The aim of showing this video was to reduce cancer fatalism, increase knowledge of colorectal cancer and increase participation in faecal occult blood testing among rural elders. The video consisted of an introduction, three scenes and a concluding segment. The video incorporated spirituality and hope into the interactive dialogues about cancer fatalism, information about colorectal cancer and demonstrations of faecal occult blood testing. The control group used the Cancer Society's video 'Colorectal Cancer: The Cancer Nobody Talks About'.

The intervention group had significantly greater decrease in cancer fatalism scores and greater increased knowledge of colorectal cancer than the control group. This study was limited and unable to generalize beyond the target population, but suggests it is possible to decrease perceptions of cancer fatalism.

Genetic screening for cancer

It is well recognized that some cancers have a genetic component. Examples include cancer of the breast, ovary and colon. To date there has been relatively little work done on attitudes towards cancer genetic testing among ethnic minorities. Honda (2003) examined awareness of genetic testing for cancer risk in the US general population. The study found that the major predictors of awareness of genetic testing were race, ethnicity, education, immigration status, health status, interaction with health professionals, cancer diagnosis and family history of cancer. He argues for looking at ways to improve quality of public knowledge of genetic testing for cancer risks. The results of this study are also supported by several other studies (e.g. Durfy *et al.* 1999; Hughes *et al.* 1997) which point to the role of ethnicity in knowledge and awareness of genetic testing for cancer. There has been little research conducted relating to how different groups understand the concept of genetic risk and their attitudes towards 'risk taking'. There is a need for future work to look at how specific ethnic groups understand and perceive the concept of risk.

Glanz *et al.* (1999) examined correlates of intention to obtain genetic counselling and colorectal gene testing among relatives who are at risk from three ethnic groups. The study looked at Caucasian, Japanese and Hawaiian patients and found high rates of interest in cancer genetic testing among all the groups similar to those found in other studies. Ethnic differences revealed a paradox between objective population risk (higher for Japanese) and greater concern (among Hawaiians). The substantial lack of awareness of family history was further researched. The authors argue that culturally sensitive education and counselling is needed for managing the high demand for personalized information about hereditary cancer risk.

There is some evidence that African American women may overestimate the impact of genetic factors and underestimate the role of social environment, physical environment and personal behaviour on breast cancer incidence (Duncan *et al.* 2001). Using a qualitative focus group design these authors found that information presented about the role of genes on breast cancer incidence may be confusing, contributing to the fact that these women generally overestimated the role of genes and underestimated the role of personal behaviour in the development of breast cancer. Women in this study appeared to lack confidence in their ability to reduce their risk, reflecting the fact that they perceived themselves to have little control over their genes. This overestimation of genetic influence on breast cancer might result from the poor literacy and numeracy in this group. Both literacy and numeracy are essential for the understanding of genetic information which is often complex and abstract and not easily accessible to the general public. These findings offer some insights into African American womens' failure to use preventive health measures. The perceived genetic causation may contribute to the cancer fatalism discussed above.

To date, there has been no work specifically examining how to communicate genetic risk in different ethnic groups. It is important to point out that the risk of developing cancer is not the same as the risk of dying with cancer. Kelly (2004) presents a good overview of the area of genetic risk assessment in oncology and describes different types of risk information: risk over time; absolute risk and comparative risk. In particular she argues that women often have difficulty hearing or absorbing risk information, that this information is more likely to be useful if presented with a time frame and in terms of absolute risk.

Summary

The role of cultural factors in the prevention of and screening for cancer has been discussed above. Although cultural beliefs such as fatalism are important in this respect, other more pragmatic factors such as language, availability, accessibility and appointment systems may be responsible for the poor uptake of screening in some cultural groups. Increasing rates of screening involves more than translating information into the particular language of a specific cultural group. It involves an in-depth understanding of attitudes about illness and its prevention and includes issues of perceived control. As will be discussed later, medical decision making in some ethnic groups is made within a family context. Due attention must be given to family systems of authority and communication in planning any screening programme.

Health education programmes need to focus on modifying beliefs and attitudes about cancer. Representatives from a given culture should be involved in consultations and may act as 'culture brokers'. There is a need to adapt messages on screening, diagnosis and treatment to the local community's ways of thinking. Screening methods must be ethnically and culturally based to overcome cultural barriers. One American project, the *Witness Project*, was developed taking into account African American misconceptions about breast cancer (a White woman's disease, a fatal disease with a stigma attached) and has resulted in an increased number of African American women getting a mammogram. In this programme culturally appropriate role models (witness role models) who had survived cancer 'witnessed' or talked about their cancer experiences with other African American women addressing the fatalistic view. These survivors both demonstrated that cancer is not a death sentence and also, by publicly discussing it, helped remove the 'stigmatization' of cancer (Bailey *et al.* 2000).

Further reading

Glanz, K., Rimer, B., Lewis, F. *et al.* (2002) *Health Behaviour and Health Education: Theory, Research and Practice*. San Francisco, CA: Jossey Bass.

Hahn, R. (1999) *Anthropology in Public Health: Bridging Differences in Culture and Society*. New York: Oxford University Press.

Naidoo, J. and Wills, J. (2000) *Health Promotion: Foundations for Practice*. Edinburgh: Balliere Tindall.

World Cancer Research Fund/American Institute for Cancer Research (1997) *Food, Nutrition and the Prevention of Cancer: A Global Perspective*. London: WCRF/AICR.

3 Communicating the diagnosis and cancer communication

A major aspect of working with cancer patients and their families involves communication. Good communication is essential at all stages of the cancer journey, from screening and diagnosis to palliative care. Communication involves more than translation. Cultural groups differ not only in the languages they use but also in the types of information they find acceptable and unacceptable (for instance, the giving of bad news) and in the ways in which this information is transmitted both verbally and non-verbally. This chapter examines three aspects of cancer communication: cross-cultural communication, breaking bad news and informed consent.

Communication always occurs within a cultural context (Moore and Butow 2004). It is only recently that the issue of culture as a context in cancer communication has been empirically studied and evaluated (Surbone and Zwitter 1997). As Moore and Spiegel (2004) point out, different forms of communication might enhance hope and positive expectations of patients and their families. Although far from proven, the beliefs and expectations of patients may significantly affect the course of their illness, both physically and psychologically. It is now well recognized that different beliefs and expectations produce different effects on bodily function. For instance, clinical analgesia depends both on the physiological action of the treatment and on the expectations of the clinician and patient. Placebo effects are relevant to clinician-patient communication and this provides one area for fruitful future research (Hahn 1997; Chvetzoff and Tannock 2003).

There is some evidence that good communication is associated with better psychological outcome in cancer. For instance, Butow *et al.* in an Australian study (1996) found psychological adjustment in cancer patients to be related to quality of doctor discussion about cancer treatment options, but *not* about the diagnosis of cancer and its implications. Other studies indicate a positive relationship between effective communication and patient satisfaction, reduced psychological morbidity, enhanced health outcomes and reduced clinician burnout (Fallowfield *et al.* 1995; Kearney 1997; Christakis 2000; Bredart *et al.* 2003; Zacharia *et al.* 2003). The interpretations of patients and their expectations influence how they feel, what they understand and how they adhere to treatment afterwards (Horwitz and Horwitz 1993).

By contrast, poor communication may deprive patients of hope and result in consequently poorer prognosis as the person feels unable to cope and has no expectation that any change will possibly help. There is some emerging evidence that low socio-economic status impacts adversely on clinician-patient communication and this in turn might influence negatively the psychological prognosis in cancer patients (Sen 1997).

Problems in cross-cultural communication

Beyond linguistic differences, there are several potential problems which might arise during consultation with ethnic minority groups. Communication with patients directly about various aspects of illness may be difficult for doctors and other health professionals working among ethnic minority groups. For instance, due to cultural taboos, it may be difficult to talk about bodily functions through an interpreter, especially if it is a male member of the community and therefore history taking among ethnic minorities by doctors may be inadequate due to a mutual lack of understanding.

Another communication problem relates to stereotyping. There is a growing literature which suggests that health professionals do stereotype patients (see Geiger 2001) and this stereotyping may result in worse treatments for ethnic minority patients. Health professionals must have a good knowledge of the various common diseases among ethnic minority groups. Lack of knowledge might result in 'diagnostic stereotyping'. It is easy to put down the symptoms, such as weight loss in South Asians, to diabetes or tuberculosis and miss a serious diagnosis of cancer due to 'cultural diagnostic stereotyping'.

Patients who have recently arrived from abroad have often experienced a different healthcare system and have different expectations from the health professional. In some cultures it may be the norm for patients to see a number of physicians or specialists for opinions, rather than one doctor. This may result in the health professional believing that the patient has little faith in them. There may be conflicts between the patient's explanatory models and the doctor's explanatory models of illness. Explanations that patients bring, for instance beliefs about possession by spirits, may be relatively inaccessible to the health professional, trained according to a biomedical model. They may be reluctant therefore to expose their beliefs to the scrutiny of a health professional. Alternatively, patients may hold that it is not their role to tell the doctor what they believe and not the professional's role to ask. In many cultures it is not acceptable for the patients to present their thoughts about their health to a health professional.

Non-verbal communication

Health professionals and patients may misinterpret each other in terms of non-verbal communication. There may be differences between cultures in gestures, touch, proximity and head and body movement. In some cultures looking the other person in the eye is a sign of honesty, in others it is a sign of disrespect, particularly between gender or age groups. Para-verbal communication includes politeness convention, how information is delivered, degrees of directness, tone of voice, stress in words, phrases, pace and the use of silence (Fuller 2003). Politeness conventions may vary across different language groups. The words please and thank you occur less commonly in some language groups, particularly South Asian. Because of this, patients from these groups may be perceived as abrupt or rude by health professionals. Afro-Caribbean, West African and South Asian language speakers tend to be more direct than English speakers. This fact might make English speakers appear to be more deceitful to these groups than they really are. There may be differences in tone, stress, pace and use of silence, which can lead to misinterpretations of motive and might influence whether information is credible and what action should be taken.

Even where language is shared, there may be significant problems with communication. Practical and clinical issues might be difficult to deal with while psychosocial issues or information sharing may be extremely difficult. Health professionals, because they are concentrating on understanding and being understood, can lose basic communication skills, which might encourage the patient to relax.

Facilitating communication

There are a number of ways of facilitating communication with different ethnic groups (see Fuller 2003). It is important to keep an even tone, not to speed up delivery and not to shout. As the consultation proceeds, it is important to signal any change of subject to the patient, especially if he or she finds it difficult to understand and is hanging on to one thread of the conversation. Confirmation that the information is understood must be obtained.

Communication may be facilitated in a number of ways: by using pictures, diagrams or mime. For instance pictures can help health professionals communicate about parts of the body. Most people have access to someone in their community who can translate. There are a number of health promotion leaflets available for each community written in the vernacular language. It is important to remember that some people, especially older people, may be illiterate in the language of their community.

When patient and doctor speak different languages, unless the doctor is proficient in the language of his patients, they will need interpreters. Feeland and Parkman (1995) have drawn attention to the disadvantages of using friends and relatives for interpreting and in particular the importance of not using children who lack the emotional and cognitive maturity to assume the responsibility of interpreting conversations between patients and professionals. In particular, details of bodily function and dysfunction are considered private and unsuitable subjects of discussion by them.

Interpreters may be informal, perhaps a family member or friend or bilingual health worker, or a formal interpreter who may be trained specifically to work in a healthcare setting. Using textual analysis, there is evidence that informal interpreters are more likely to make errors than professional interpreters. These errors include deletions and insertions which may distort the meaning of the interpreting communication. They often impose their own agenda on the consultation, rather than that of the patient and they may be reluctant to bring up certain 'taboo' topics. By contrast, professional interpreters will generally have received adequate training in relation to the healthcare context of the NHS.

Types of interpretation

Most attempts to overcome language barriers involve consecutive interpretation which uses a pause while speech content is delivered in a second language. Consecutive interpreting can be delivered by a physically present interpreter or by a remote interpreter using a telephone line. Attention must be paid to seating arrangements. A triangular seating arrangement is most appropriate since it allows health professionals to see and clearly communicate with both the interpreter and the patient. It is important to try and speak directly to the patient. The use of jargon and figures of speech should be avoided and health professionals should speak a sentence or two before passing on to the interpreter to interpret. Particular care is required for explaining procedures or the details of medicines and arrangements for follow-up and review. Important information may need to be repeated and written material given in the patient's language. It is vital to ask the patient at the end of the consultation if there is anything else they want to say or ask. In the USA there have been attempts to explore the use of simultaneous interpreting, using headsets in a similar way to their use in multilingual international conference settings.

In the USA telephone interpreting is common. It involves both patient and professional using hands-free phones with an interpreter on the telephone line. This service may result in loss of potentially supportive face-to-face contact. However, it may prevent issues of embarrassment or concerns about confidentiality because interpreters are unlikely to come from the same locality as the patient. Jones and Gill (2003) provide a good overview of the use of interpreters in primary care and should be consulted for further discussion of this topic.

Communicating the diagnosis of cancer

Box 3.1

Mohammad, a 70-year-old man from Pakistan, developed carcinoma of the bowel which was diagnosed at a late stage. His family accompanied him to his consultation with the gastroenterologist. They told the physician not to disclose the diagnosis of cancer to him, since they believed that he was unable to withstand this. The physician 'colluded' with this opinion. He was finally admitted into a local hospice. A major conflict ensued. The hospice staff were keen to tell him what was wrong with him, arguing that he would find out in any case. The family were against this. They argued that it was for the family to know but not for the patient. Mohammad died shortly after. It was uncertain whether he really knew his diagnosis.

Attitudes towards informing patients that they have cancer or that they are dying have changed since the mid-1970s both in the USA and UK. An early study of people's wishes to be told whether they had cancer indicated that they themselves preferred to be told but were less in favour of recommending that others in a similar position should be informed (Kelly and Trleson 1950). Oken's (1961) American study documented that 90 per cent of responding physicians preferred not to tell patients the diagnosis. When this study was repeated in 1979 (Novack *et al.* 1979), 97 per cent of responding physicians indicated a preference for telling the cancer patients.

There is no evidence that honest communication causes detrimental effects and little evidence for the fear that these patients are more likely to commit suicide (Hinton 1991). Centeno-Cortes and Nun-Olarte (1994) found no increase in perceived symptoms of anxiety, despair, sadness, depression, insomnia or fear in a group of informed patients compared to uninformed patients. In this study there were clear benefits in those who had been told – 75 per cent of informed patients were able to share their concerns about the illness and its consequences with their relatives, whereas only 25 per cent of those who were uninformed were able to do so. In fact, one might argue that most dying people have some awareness of their own situation and this has been found to be the case even in children (Hinton 1963; Waechter 1971). There is little evidence supporting the contention that terminally ill patients, who have not been told the truth of their situation, die happily in blissful ignorance. The dying person witnesses their deteriorating body, fatigue and reduction in ability to function which indicate that they are dying. Relatives, friends and healthcare professionals give out non-verbal clues as to what is happening. There is however evidence to support the fact that honest communication is what the majority of patients want and expect in order to plan and make decisions about the place of death, put their affairs in order, say goodbyes, forgive old adversaries and be protected from embarking on unpleasant and futile therapies.

Failure to disclose information may create difficulties in the doctor/patient relationship. Fallowfield (1997), in a paper entitled 'Truth sometimes hurts but deceit hurts more', notes that healthcare professionals often censor their information-giving to patients in an attempt to protect them from potentially hurtful, sad or bad news. This desire to shield patients from the reality of their situation usually creates even greater difficulty for patients, their relatives and friends and other members of the healthcare team. There are many reasons why healthcare professionals may not wish to communicate openly. They may believe that the patient will ask, if they really wish to know. The patient may assume the doctors will tell them everything, they may be too scared to ask, or the patient may try to make it easier for the doctor and therefore not ask questions.

Disclosure in modern Western societies

Seale (1998) reports how, in two national surveys in 1969 and 1987 in the UK, the proportion of dying people reported to have certainly known that they were dying rose from 16 per cent to 44 per cent for those with cancer. This trend towards open disclosure in modern Western societies has continued throughout the 1990s. As Seale, Addington-Hall and McCarthy (1997: 447) point out, 'A preference for open awareness of dying is now established in terminal care settings and among the general population in the UK, USA and other Anglophone countries.' This shift in disclosure is likely to have resulted from a number of factors, both medical and social: improvements in therapeutic success, changing societal attitudes and in the USA, legislation enforcing the patient's right to 'informed consent'.

Despite the perceived trend towards 'open disclosure' of the patient's terminal prognosis, Field and Copp (1999) suggest that there is currently a progression towards 'conditional disclosure', in which disclosure appears over a period of time and that health workers moderate and back away from automatic disclosure of a terminal prognosis. They cite a number of studies to support this contention.

Taylor (1988) observed Canadian physicians in a breast cancer clinic. Although these physicians told women that they had breast cancer, the majority evaded or dissimulated when discussing the likely prognosis and treatment choices with patients, immediately following their disclosure to the patient that a cancerous lump had been found. In only 10 per cent of the 118 consultations that she observed, was there 'effective communication in disclosure'. Similarly, Miyaji (1993) in the USA found that physicians appeared to be open in their disclosure of diagnosis, but less forthcoming in their disclosure of a terminal prognosis. The majority stated that they would respond to what the patient wanted to know about diagnosis and prognosis. That is, the amount of information actually given was dependent upon the doctor's assessment of what the patient wanted, and needed, to know. Individual doctors had their own ways of disclosing information based upon one or more of five main principles:

- the respect for truth;
- the patients' rights;
- the duty to inform;
- maintaining hope;
- the sanctity of the individual contract between patient and doctor.

In an interview study in the UK of general medical practitioners, Field (1998) found that doctors tempered, delayed and modified full and open disclosure of terminal prognosis to their cancer patients and modified their initial statements that they were 'open and honest' in their communications with terminally ill patients. Hence these doctors retained control over information and its disclosure despite their stated commitment to an ideology of 'open awareness'.

These studies indicate a retraction from the full and frank disclosure of terminal prognosis advocated by proponents of the open awareness movement of the late 1960s–1980s. Similarly, specialists in palliative care also appear to have adopted a more traditional approach to disclosing terminal prognosis, although direct evidence for this is lacking. Overall, there has been a move from closed awareness to open awareness and partially back to conditional awareness. This appears to be a more pragmatic and responsive pattern of communication. It seems that dying patients are not constant in their emotional and cognitive responses to the likelihood of imminent death and there may now be a greater acceptance by health workers of the advantages of patient denial at various times as they approach death.

Research on disclosure, however, is problematic and there are a number of difficult issues in looking at disclosure empirically. First, it is difficult to compare studies using varying methodologies, ranging from quantitative surveys of physicians' attitudes, retrospective qualitative studies of patients' experiences, surrogate accounts of carers, qualitative semistructured interviews with hospice patients and qualitative interviews with physicians. Second, it may be difficult to interpret evidence relating to putatatively terminal diagnoses and prognoses. Third, there are severe problems of ascertaining patients' knowledge and awareness about their death, in that patients may not be open about their beliefs and feelings to researchers and may be unwilling to discuss this topic. Researchers may experience difficulty asking about such sensitive topics, which are taboo in Western society.

The ethics of disclosing the truth

There are three main ethical influences which affect Western physicians' truth-telling practices (Beauchamp and Childress 2001; Dein and Thomas 2002). They are:

1 Consequentialism: a label affixed to theories holding that actions are right or wrong according to the balance of their good or bad consequences;
2 Belief in patient rights and autonomy. There is an assumption that the patient is able to determine his or her treatment. The patient can act autonomously as an individual in his or her own right;
3 The sense of professional duty or responsibility.

Each of the above may vary cross-culturally. For instance, in some cultures concern for the patient's welfare and physicians not doing anything which threatens a patient's well-being override principles of autonomy. Approaches to truth telling in the West are dependent on the Western understanding of individualism, where the patient is an autonomous agent and therefore responsible for decisions regarding health and entitled to involvement in therapeutic decision making (Surbone and Zwitter 1997). In many parts of the world the patient is firmly situated within an extended family which assumes the responsibility for help seeking and decision making and which shields the ill person from the truth about diagnosis and prognosis in terminal illness (Malik and Quereshi 1997; Younge et al. 1997; Pellegrino 1998).

Blackhall et al. (1995) examined differences in the attitudes of elderly subjects from different ethnic groups (European American, African American, Korean American and Mexican American) towards disclosure of the diagnosis and prognosis of a terminal illness. Korean American and Mexican American subjects were more likely to hold a family-centred model of medical decision making than the patient autonomy model held by most of the African American and European American subjects.

Cross-cultural aspects of truth telling: the views of doctors and patients

It is recognized that cultural factors influence attitudes towards truth telling. In terms of the wish to be told a serious diagnosis, significantly fewer people in Japan than in Britain or New Zealand would wish to be told that they were dying (Charlton and Dovey 1995). At present, most physicians in the USA and Europe presume that cancer patients ought to be informed of their illness. By contrast, within countries such as Japan and Italy, it is still common for physicians and family members to conceal diagnoses of cancer, especially terminal diagnoses. The idea of open disclosure may be Anglocentric, inappropriate for certain patients (Field and Copp 1999), and may even be seen as shocking (Seale 1998). The justification for withholding information is that patients are given hope and are protected from what is considered devastating knowledge.

There is evidence that doctors' willingness for open disclosure of a life-threatening diagnosis may vary across the world. Bruera *et al.* (2000) used a postal survey to examine the attitudes and beliefs of palliative care specialists towards communication with the terminally ill in Europe, South America and Canada. Although all physicians said they would like to be told the truth about their own terminal illness, only 93 per cent of Canadian physicians, 26 per cent of European and 18 per cent of South American physicians thought that the majority of their patients would wish to know. There were similar major differences in terms of attitudes towards discussing these issues with relatives.

However, breaking bad news may not be done very well, even if physicians hold a positive attitude towards disclosure. There is evidence that clinicians often rate their skills as deficient in terms of communicating bad news to patients and relatives in both mono-ethnic and multicultural populations (Surbone and Zwitter 1997; Chambers 2000). These findings have been corroborated by audit studies which provide direct evidence of deficiencies in these areas (Gattellari *et al.* 2002). Minority groups report that health professionals often do not understand them and this might lead to them avoiding biomedical encounters until the disease is advanced, or preferring to consult clinicians deriving from their own cultural groups. A study of Greeks living in Australia indicated that they would prefer to see Greek doctors whom they perceived to make them feel less 'inferior' because of their poor language skills (Goldstein *et al.* 2002).

Disclosure among ethnic minorities in the UK

In some Asian cultures members of the family unit may withhold the truth about terminal illness from elders out of respect and a desire to protect them from harm. Spruyt's (1999) study of 18 bereaved Bangladeshi carers found that all patients were aware of the diagnosis. However, only six carers agreed that it was right to disclose because their relative had a right to the truth and so that the patient could prepare for death. They acknowledged that the openness about diagnosis brought them closer. Eight opposed disclosure because they felt that it would be weakening, destroy hope and create anxiety and depression. Firth (1997) found that for Hindus and Sikhs living in the UK, a good death was a conscious and anticipated one and advanced knowledge was considered essential to enable people to prepare spiritually and practically. However, relatives resisted this knowledge and tried to control the information on the grounds that it would upset the patient.

European traditions

Greece

Mystakidou *et al.* (1996) deployed a postal survey of a representative sample of 300 oncologists, radiotherapists and palliative care specialists, asking about the disclosure of a cancer diagnosis to patients. The study indicated that withholding the truth from cancer patients remains very common in Greece. Another Greek study (Georgaki *et al.* 2002) examined Greek nurses' attitudes towards truth-telling practices when working with cancer patients and their psychological status regarding the difficulties they face in their day-to-day communication with these patients. Although many Greek nurses believed that the patient should be informed and know their condition, lack of training in communication skills was a major obstacle to achieving this.

Italy

Gordon and Paci (1997) note that non-disclosure is common in Italy where it is considered important to maintain hope, security and tranquillity rather than a combative spirit in the face of terminal illness. They argue that it is therefore a mistake to remove hope, which 'leaves room for positive fantasy' (Gordon and Paci 1997: 1449), although the authors comment that this appears to leave little room for aggressive treatment and experimental therapies. Women with breast cancer in their study indicated that they wished to be informed of their diagnosis, but not that they were terminally ill or dying, and that they lived in fluctuating states of knowing and not knowing.

Poland

It is rare for cancer patients to receive a truthful diagnosis and prognosis in Poland (Meyza 1997). Generally, the family is informed by the physician about the diagnosis and for hospital staff, cancer still remains a 'taboo' subject. Incurable patients are often discharged home as soon as possible. Until the late 1990s, the usual practice in hospitals was to hide the diagnosis and prognosis of cancer, except in the case of patients reluctant to accept the proposed treatment. Even then, the information is restricted to naming the treatment modalities. However, a different approach is adopted in hospices, where the first information about the diagnosis comes from the staff.

Disclosure in the Judeo-Christian tradition

Religious Catholics hold that the doctor is obliged personally to inform the patient of the hopelessness of the condition, if the latter finds himself or herself in a state of mortal sin, or in need of ordering the affairs of estate. Any failure to do so involves the doctor in great sin, since it allows spiritual or material damage to occur which could have been prevented. This attitude prevails, even if such knowledge may lead to depression or endangering their life.

The attitude towards disclosure is very different in Orthodox Judaism. Based on biblical authority, Orthodox Jews hold that even when their physician realizes that his patient approaches death, he should not tell him that the death is imminent for fear he or she will give up and die (Neuberger 1998; Katz 2000; Bodell and Weng 2000). The Jewish tradition is intensely life-affirming. The question of disclosure of terminal illness thus presents an ethical dilemma. On the one hand, the Torah commands Jews to 'choose life' and the maintenance of life is a primary concern. On the other hand, not telling the patient may prevent him or her ordering their affairs and reciting the death bed confession. This dilemma is particularly acute when there is a question of withdrawing hydration from a dying person, as this involves disclosure and could also hasten death. However, Judaism does not require the total avoidance of all mention of death. In the very last stages of life it may be acceptable to disclose this information to the patient.

Resolving the ethical dilemmas of disclosure

Ethical issues may arise when immigrants from certain non-disclosure cultures encounter physicians whose practice it is to disclose bad news. Karim *et al.* (2000) point out that diagnosis of a life-threatening illness is often withheld from ethnic minority patients and staff are commonly asked to collude with families in concealing this. What should the obligations of physicians be to patients and their family members in North America and Europe, who come from countries where information disclosure about illness is not the norm? Should the health professional just go ahead and tell the patient? Or should he or she withhold this information in accordance with the patient or family's wishes? There are no simple answers to this dilemma and it is possible that over time ethical norms among minority groups may adapt to Western notions. A compromise would be to discuss in detail attitudes of the family towards truth telling and explain the normative practice. Allaying misconceptions about truth telling might allow the physician to be honest with his or her patient and may ultimately improve the doctor-patient relationship. Lee and Wu (2002), working in Singapore, have discussed the problem of family collusion and suggest several ways of dealing with it. This framework can be deployed in the UK and USA and includes:

1 Acknowledging that the family knows the patient best;
2 Establishing the reasons for withholding information from the patient;
3 Determining the cost of keeping the news from the patient;
4 Asking for permission to speak to the patient alone in order to establish what he or she wants to know, rather than force the bad news on the patient;
5 Acknowledging any identified emotional distress in the family, for example, guilt over delay in bringing their relative for treatment or anxiety about the future;
6 Reassuring the family that they will be updated with details of the conversation with the patient.

The issue of disclosure is seminal to understanding problems with informed consent now to be discussed.

Informed consent for treatment and research among ethnic minorities: ethics and cultural relativism

The Nuremberg Code (Shuster 1997), Helsinki Declaration IV (World Medical Association 2000) and the Council of International Organisations of Medical Sciences Ethical Guidelines (CIOMS 2002) emphasize the need for full disclosure, hence enabling individuals to make free and informed decisions about participating in research. It cannot be assumed that all cultures will understand consent in the same way. Understanding of informed consent depends on notions of autonomy, doctor/patient relationships and decision making in the family. As discussed above, in many non-Western cultures it is the family rather than the individual patient that makes decisions about treatment. In some cultural groups it is customary for a husband to make decisions for his wife and this extends to participation in research. Women are therefore not autonomous in these groups. Issues of coercion may arise in cultures in which doctors have a very high status and are not questioned. Patients may consent on account of the belief that it is unacceptable to disagree with the doctor or his or her team. There may be differing cultural expectations concerning the roles of both clinicians and patients, which indirectly influence types of communications which occur in the clinical encounter. For instance, patients of Chinese descent generally hold great respect for the clinician's expertise. Any ambivalence or uncertainty in presenting the diagnosis or treatment recommendations might be viewed as reflecting a lack of expertise (Huang *et al.* 1999) and the suggestion of active patient participation in decision making may be interpreted as incompetence. Past experiences of research misdemeanours may militate against participation in research. At the extreme, some patients may see informed consent as a waiver for liability reminding them of past events, such as that which occurred in Tuskagee, where experiments on syphilis treatment were carried out on African Americans without their consent.

The cross-cultural application of informed consent procedures, to say the least, is problematic. Each group has its own conception of ethics, based on its culture, which must be individually understood by researchers. The question therefore arises as to whether ethical systems derived from Western cultures should be applied to all cultures. According to a cultural relativistic position different societies have different moral codes. There is no one objective standard to judge one societal ethical code as better than another. Notions of right and wrong are defined by the culture in which they occur. From this perspective Western ethical principles have no privileged status (Rachels 2002). In some cultures, ethics is more a fluid concept that requires constant re-examination and redefinition and informed consent is viewed and implemented as an ongoing process. This implies that consent must be asked for and given at almost every step of the research process to assure that it is valid (Bergum 1989). It is argued here, however, that it is possible to modify existing Western derived informed consent procedures for some members of ethnic minority groups, rather than adopting a completely relativistic stance, which accepts that each group must adopt its unique ethical principles including those relating to consent. If one accepts ethical relativism, the theory that morality is relative to the norms of one's culture, there can be no common framework for resolving moral disputes.

Some members of ethnic minority groups in the UK are unable to read or write, even in their own language (or their own language has no written form, such as Syhleti). This renders the filling in of consent forms difficult or impossible. In cultures whereby contracts are made verbally, asking for a signature may imply mistrust and cause offence. However despite these difficulties, standard procedures still require written consent. More specifically, there may be significant levels of 'health illiteracy' which may prevent individuals from learning about and participating in research. An individual's ability to read and comprehend health-related materials, such as medication instructions and informed consent forms, may be substantially weaker than their general literacy. Illiteracy must never be taken to mean that a potential participant is unable to comprehend complex information, just that it must be presented in a different form. Problems of illiteracy are often confounded by lack of education which may be more important than ethnicity in determining participation in and understanding of clinical trials (Hussain-Gambles *et al.* 2004).

Problems in implementing informed consent in ethnic minority groups may be addressed in a number of ways: simplifying and making the consent forms more readable; spending more time with participants explaining the consent process; and providing more information about the project in order to enhance understanding among those who may lack it. One possibility could be to write a more detailed information sheet. To ensure that comprehension is adequate, researchers could use a questionnaire or interview to ensure that participants have acquired this information before consent is given. In illiterate groups, information may be provided visually, for example by using videos or illustrations, which might enhance the comprehension and retention of concepts (Wood *et al.* 2001). Researchers may require the consent of a community leader before being permitted to engage in research with this community; however this does not compromise the need to obtain individual informed consent. Before consent can be freely given, issues of disclosure need to be addressed as discussed above. For a fuller discussion on this topic see Dein and Bhai (2005).

Summary

Good communication is essential in oncology but working with ethnic minority patients may present certain difficulties. There is a need for oncology health professionals to have knowledge of the different cultural patterns of communication among the populations in which they work. This is an aspect of cultural competence which will be discussed at length in the last chapter. Communication requires knowledge of family structures, power relationships within the family and their influences on medical decision making.

Future research should focus on culture specific patterns of communication in relation to cancer. Relevant areas for future research include: attitudes towards disclosure in different cultural groups; culture specific modes of doctor-patient communication (both verbal and non verbal); cultural aspects of medical decision making; the establishment of guidelines for informed consent in different groups; and the influence of different types of communication on psychological outcomes in cancer patients.

Further reading

Faulkner, A. and Maguire, P. (1994) *Talking to Cancer Patients and their Relatives.* Oxford: Oxford University Press.

Kai, J. (2003) *Ethnicity, Health, and Primary Care.* Oxford: Oxford University Press.

Moore, R. and Spiegel, D. (2004) *Cancer, Culture and Communication.* New York: Kluwer Academic/Plenum Publishers.

4 The cultural response to cancer, coping and the role of religion and spirituality

The response to negative life events is highly influenced by the cultural context and can range from extreme stoicism to severe depression. There is evidence that culture may determine the way in which sufferers respond to cancer, both in terms of psychological and physical symptoms, including pain. Knowledge of these varied responses is of importance to health professionals who, without this cultural knowledge, might judge the response in individuals from one cultural group to be abnormal, when in fact it is culturally appropriate.

Common reactions to cancer include denial, anger, depression and anxiety. Anger may be directed to doctors (who are blamed for picking up the cancer late) or sometimes towards God or another religious figure. Those diagnosed with cancer often ask the question 'why me?' At the same time, they are angry when no answer is forthcoming (see Box 4.1).

Adjustment problems occur frequently in people with cancer (Barraclough 1999; Chochinov and Breitbart 2000). Anxiety is the most common form of distress. This may increase at particular times: at initial investigation of suspicious symptoms; at the time of diagnosis; when primary treatment ends; at disease recurrence; when a bad prognosis is disclosed; and in the terminal phase of illness (Dein 2003). There are many possible coping responses. Common responses include fighting spirit, helplessness, fatalism, anxious preoccupation, emotional suppression and avoidance. It is known that poor adjustment is related to a previous psychiatric history, lack of support, inability to accept physical changes, lack of involvement in satisfying activities, low expectation that the treatment will be effective or a previous bad experience of cancer in the family. Emotional suppression and avoidance are associated with poorer coping responses (Massie *et al.* 1994).

Box 4.1

A 17-year-old man, a practising Hindu, became angry with God when his father developed terminal colon cancer. He asked his physician why his father had developed the cancer in the first place and why he was suffering so much. He felt it was very unfair that he had been good throughout his life and was ill, while criminals, who did nothing good, lived a long life. The son expressed anger towards God for allowing him to become ill and for not answering his prayers.

He had sought the advice of a *pandit* who told him that all illness was a trial and that his father would get through the test and recover. This blatantly was not the case. His father's illness had caused him to lose faith in God and stop praying. The son asked whether his father had been bad in a previous life and was suffering in this life on account of this, a belief consistent with the Hindu notion of *karma*. His only consolation was that his father might be reborn into a much better life, since he held reincarnation to be a strong possibility.

It is important to be aware of cultural and religious differences when looking at patterns of adjustment to cancer. There is evidence that Western cultures use different coping strategies than individuals from non-Western cultures (Barg and Gullatte 2001). These differences derive from variations in basic values and cultural norms, relating to reliance on the family and others for social support and the value of individual, as opposed to group, coping efforts. Some Asian American groups, for example, tend not to ruminate on upsetting thoughts, thinking that reticence or avoidance is better than outward expression. They place a greater emphasis on suppression of affect (Kleinman 1970; Hsu 1971), with some tending first to rely on themselves to cope with distress (Narikiyo and Kameoka 1992). African Americans tend to adopt an active approach in facing personal problems rather than avoiding them (Broman 1996). They are more likely than Whites to handle distress on their own (Sussman *et al.* 1987). They also appear to rely more on spirituality to help them cope with adversity and symptoms of mental illness (Broman 1996; Neighbors *et al.* 1998; Cooper-Patrick *et al.* 1999).

In some cultures there is an emphasis on stoicism and the acceptance of adversity. For instance, it has been reported that Vietnamese patients are often stoical (La Borde 2004). Uba (1992) points out how Southeast Asian refugees in the USA value stoicism and view suffering and illness as part of life and thus may not seek medical care until later stages of disease.

There may be difficulty in detecting distress in patients from some cultural or religious groups. There are several reasons for this: varying expressions of distress; difficulty in judging the patient's demeanour; and misunderstanding behaviour which may seem abnormal in one culture and normal in another. Cultures may differ in their norms of self-disclosure or privacy regarding subjective experiences. This may influence their willingness to answer questions about this type of experience (Bullinger *et al.* 1993). This might render research in cross-cultural emotional reactions difficult.

The cultural shaping of depression

The ways in which emotions are experienced and expressed is dependent on the cultural context. Anthropologists have argued that emotional experience is not precultural, but preeminently cultural, and is shaped by indigenous models of the self and social interaction (Lutz 1988). This emphasis on the social construction of emotion does not imply a complete denial of biological aspects. There is an evolving literature suggesting that various emotional states, such as anxiety and depression, are highly subject to cultural influence, which shapes both their experience and their expression (Kleinman 1980; Littlewood and Dein 2000).

The cultural variation in somatization – the presentation of emotional states as physical symptoms – has been widely discussed in the literature (Silveira and Ebrahim 1995; Goh *et al.* 1996). In relation to depression, Ramirez *et al.* (1991) found evidence that there were cultural differences in the frequency with which certain manifestations of this emotional state presented. These included differences in the frequency of somatization, guilt feelings and suicidal ideation. They point out that somatization of depressive illness is more common in the non-European than European cultures. Within some cultures, such as the Chinese, somatization may be the culturally sanctioned manner of expressing affective symptoms (Kleinmann and Kleinmann 1985). However, somatization may be a Western conceptualization, foreign to other cultures: 'Placing mind and body in separate disciplinary domains is inconceivable in the Asian world view' (Kagawa-Singer *et al.* 1997).

Other symptoms related to depression, such as hopelessness and guilt, may be culturally specific. For instance, Krause (1989) administered the GHQ (General Health Questionnaire) to Punjabis in the UK and found that questions regarding hope resulted in defensive laughter about the stupidity of the question because 'it is not for us to have hope'. In some groups, such as Muslims, there may be difficulty with the word 'depression' because feeling depressed may show a lack of respect for Allah (Goh *et al.* 1996).

Are there differences in the reaction to and the ways of coping with cancer in different ethnic groups?

To date, there has been relatively little ethnographic research specifically examining cultural differences in the reactions to, and ways of coping with, cancer in different cultural groups. Much of the work has concentrated on ethnic minority women in America. There is little data specifically relating to the UK. There is some evidence, however, suggesting that rates of psychological morbidity may vary cross-culturally. Mexican Americans, for instance, have been found to experience higher than average rates of fatalism, anxiety and depression after the diagnosis, compared with other American groups (Meyerowitz *et al.* 1998).

A study by Kagawa Singer *et al.* (1997) compared the response to breast cancer among Asian American and White American women. The study hypothesized that Asian American women would express emotions somatically. Contrary to the hypothesis, somatization did not appear to be the dominant form of symptom presentation for Asian American women, regardless of level of acculturation. There were, however, differences in help-seeking behaviour between the two groups. Asian American women sought professional assistance for psychosocial problems at a significantly lower rate than Anglo women.

Spencer *et al.*'s (1999) study examines psychosocial well-being and concerns about breast cancer in a cross sectional example of Hispanic, non-Hispanic, White and Black women. This study found elevated concerns and emotional distress among Hispanic women. Black women reported fewer concerns than Hispanic or non-Hispanic White women and reported less distress than Hispanic women. African American women with stage II and recurrent breast cancer were found to be more likely than White women to use repressive coping styles, as opposed to active coping styles, regardless of educational level (Hunt 2001).

Culver *et al.* (2002) examined coping and distress in African American, Hispanic and non-Hispanic White women with early stage breast cancer. African American women reported the lowest levels of distress, particularly before surgery, and fewer depression symptoms. Hispanic women reported the highest levels of self-destructive thoughts. Non-Hispanic White women commonly resorted to humour as a way of coping. The use of venting was common among Hispanics. African American and Hispanic women reported more religious coping than non-Hispanic White women. This is consistent with other data, which suggest that African Americans use more religious coping than non-Hispanic White people.

The importance of spirituality was emphasized in a study of 66 African American women in the south eastern United States (Henderson *et al.* 2003), which looked at specific coping mechanisms used by women with a diagnosis of breast cancer. The coping strategies described by these women included relying on prayer, avoiding negative people, developing a positive attitude, having a will to live, and receiving support from family, friends and support networks. Overall spirituality played a major role in coping with their cancer. It has been suggested that the use of spiritual and religious coping may be more common in African Americans since they face more discrimination and prejudice in general, and specifically in relation to healthcare, therefore they often turn to God and to the church (Musick *et al.* 1998).

Ell and Nishimoto (1989) found a number of differences in coping between non-Hispanic, White and Hispanic (Puerto Rican) cancer patients. Hispanics tended to have more difficulty accepting a cancer diagnosis than the other groups and were more likely to rely on religion than the Whites. For the Hispanic groups spirituality is often expressed through organized religion, particularly Roman Catholicism, and the family is an important conduit of expression of religious and spiritual activity (Gibson *et al.* 2004).

The emotional reaction to cancer may be influenced by the ability to deal with uncertainty and this in itself may vary with culture. There is some evidence that ethnic factors may determine the psychological response to uncertainty in some cancers. Germino *et al.* (1998) examined uncertainty in prostate cancer in White and African American men and their family caregivers. For both groups uncertainty was inversely related to psychological distress, i.e. the more uncertainty, the greater the psychological distress. In this study there were significant ethnic differences in the relationship of uncertainty to a number of quality of life and coping variables. The study suggests that the experience of uncertainty related to cancer and its treatment is influenced by the cultural perspective of patients and their families.

Ethnicity and cancer pain

Helman (2001) notes how each culture and social group has its own unique 'language of distress': its own idiom by which sick individuals make other people aware of their suffering. This idiom may be verbal or non-verbal and depends on, as Landy (1977: 313) puts it, 'whether their culture values or disvalues the display of emotional expression and response to injury'. Pain is a significant symptom in many cancer patients and occurs in 30 per cent of patients in those newly diagnosed and in 75 per cent of those with advanced disease (Cherny 1998). About 90 per cent of cancer pain can be well controlled using already known principles of pain management and following referral to specialist centres most of the remaining pain may be controlled.

There is an extensive medical literature indicating that people belonging to racial and ethnic minority groups in the USA, on average, are significantly less likely to receive treatment for pain, including opioid therapy, compared to non-Hispanic White people (Cleeland *et al.* 1997; Bonham 2001; Paice and O'Donnell 2004). The majority of studies conducted to date have found some disparity in pain treatment. Black and Hispanic American patients are more likely to be under-treated for pain than White patients. For instance, Cleeland *et al.* (1994) found that outpatients with cancer pain attending clinics which served ethnic minority patients were three times more likely to be under-medicated with analgesics than patients in clinics which did not serve ethnic and racial minority patients. A second study by Cleeland *et al.* (1997) indicated that ethnic minority patients received inadequate doses of analgesia compared with non-minority patients. There is evidence that minority populations such as African Americans receive inadequate end-of-life care, including poor pain control (Crawley 2002).

Several questions arise in relation to pain treatment for minority patients. Do different ethnic groups express pain in different ways? Are there significant differentials in pain thresholds in different groups? Why are some ethnic groups denied adequate analgesia? Barriers to adequate pain control can be attributed to three factors: to healthcare professionals, to patients, or to the healthcare system which may be institutionally racist (Paice and O'Donnell 2004). The most obvious barrier relates to the fact that some physicians hold stereotypical views of racial minorities that causes them to under-estimate pain in these patient populations. One belief is that some ethnic groups do not experience pain to the same degree as White people. Classic studies on pain and group membership have indicated how ethnic norms for appropriate pain behaviour influence pain perception, interpretation and response (Zborowski 1952; Zola 1966). In Zola's study there were significant differences in the public presentation of pain between ethnic groups; Irish catholic Americans were found to be more stoical about pain than Italian or Jewish Americans.

Other stereotypes might present barriers to adequate analgesia. The healthcare system may be racist. There is some evidence that non-minorities believe that minorities 'live off welfare, are more prone to violence, are less intelligent and lazy' (Davis and Smith 1990). This might cause health professionals to believe that minority patients are not capable of being involved in medical decision making, including looking after their own pain.

Poor communication between patients and physicians may lead to worse treatment for ethnic minority patients. This may simply be a lack of familiarity of comfort level or it may manifest in a sense of being not understood. A small degree of discomfort, or inability to accurately read verbal cues or body language, can contribute to a less engaged relationship between physician and patient. This disengagement may have a significant impact on treatment. Physicians may be more likely to pay greater attention to and be more engaged with the treatment of patients with whom they feel they have a closer connection.

Barriers to adequate pain control may derive from patients. Socio-economic status can also significantly influence communication. Those patients who have few economic resources are known to receive poorer medical treatment in general. Those who are more economically disadvantaged may possess a lower level of education and this may relate to difficulties in pain communication. Patients may be reluctant to report pain for fear of jeopardizing aggressive disease orientated treatments and not being perceived as a 'good' patient (Paice and O'Donnell 2004). They may be reluctant to take medications for fear of addiction or stigmatization and concerns about side effects. There is evidence that African American and Mexican American patients hold suffering to be associated with dignity and therefore minimize discomfort or report later in the illness course (Bowling 1995).

Overcoming these disparities in cancer pain treatment is thus an urgent priority. It will require collaboration between oncologists and medical anthropologists to further explore barriers to treatment and how they might be overcome.

Religion and spirituality

The terms 'spirituality' and 'religion' are often used interchangeably. However, for many people they have different meanings. Religion can be defined as a specific set of beliefs and practices associated with an organized group, whereas spirituality may be defined as an individual sense of peace, connection to others and beliefs about the meaning of life (Dein 2004b, c). Although spirituality might be expressed through organized religion, it may also be expressed in other ways. Some patients might consider themselves both religious and spiritual, whereas others may call themselves spiritual but not religious. Cancer challenges a patient's beliefs or religious values and can result in high levels of spiritual stress. They may lose faith in God or see their cancer as a punishment from God. On the other hand, spiritual beliefs may facilitate coping with cancer.

A knowledge of the role that religion and spirituality play in the patient's life may enable health professionals to understand how religious and spiritual beliefs affect the patient's response to cancer diagnosis and decisions about treatment. In relation to this, there has been recent discussion in the palliative care literature about the use of spiritual assessment tools (e.g. Puchalski 1999, Box 4.2). Broadly, this spiritual assessment should look at a number of areas: religious denomination; beliefs or philosophy of life; important spiritual practices or rituals; participation in the religious community; use of prayer and meditation; and loss of faith. Health professionals may also need to bring up issues of death, dying and the afterlife. They may, however, be reluctant to ask questions in this area since they might believe that a patient's religious/spiritual views are private or they may not feel competent to deal with these issues. The American Academy of Hospice and

Box 4.2 Spiritual assessment tools: Taking a spiritual history (Puchalski 1999)

What is your faith or belief?
Do you consider yourself spiritual or religious?
What things do you believe in that give you meaning to your life?
Is your faith or belief important in your life?
What influence does it have on how you take care of yourself?
How have your beliefs influenced your behaviour during this illness?
What role do your beliefs play in regaining your health?
Are you part of a religious or spiritual community?
Is this of support to you and how?
Is there a person or group of people you really love or who are really important to you?
How would you like me, your healthcare provider to address these issues in your healthcare?

Palliative Medicine has put together several excellent teaching videos (for instance *How We Die*) to help facilitate these discussions.

Patients can expect health professionals to respect their religious and spiritual beliefs and concerns. Those who are religious or spiritual might expect referral to the appropriate spiritual religious resources. Health professionals should respect the patient's use of religious coping during the illness and encourage patients to speak with their clergy or spiritual leader.

Do religion and spirituality facilitate coping with cancer?

The study of the relation between spirituality and health is at an early stage. However, it appears that resort to religion or spiritual coping may be a common and effective way of dealing with the stresses of cancer. In an American study of 103 women with breast cancer (Johnson and Spilka 1991), the authors found that 85 per cent reported that religion helped them cope with their cancer. The authors note 'It is evident that religion is an extremely important resource for these breast cancer patients' (p. 21). Carver *et al.* (1993), in a prospective cohort study of women with breast cancer, found acceptance, positive reframing and the use of religion were the most common coping strategies. In a study of women with gynaecological cancers (Roberts *et al.* 1997), 76 per cent of informants reported that religion had a 'serious place' in their lives. Similarly, those with lung cancer spontaneously reported religious faith and family support to be the most frequently used support systems (Ginsberg *et al.* 1995).

There is some suggestion that spiritual and religious coping is associated with improved quality of life – lower levels of anxiety, depression, hostility and discomfort. The sense of isolation, often experienced by cancer patients, may be reduced. Adjustment to the effects of cancer and its treatment might be improved and there may be enhanced ability to enjoy life during cancer treatment and a sense of personal growth may occur as a result of living with cancer (Kaczorowski 1989; Carpenter *et al.* 1999; Nelson *et al.* 2002). Musick *et al.* (1998) suggest that, among African Americans, religious activities may buffer against depression.

Specific characteristics of strong religious beliefs, including hope, optimism, freedom from regret and life satisfaction, have also been associated with improved adjustment in patients with cancer (Weisman and Worden 1977; Pargament 1997; Laubmeier *et al.* 2004). Prayer or other religious activities may sustain hope in those with cancer (Mickley *et al.* 1992; Raleigh 1992; Roberts *et al.* 1997). Spiritual well-being, particularly a sense of meaning and peace, is significantly related to the ability of cancer patients to continue to enjoy life, despite high levels of pain and fatigue (Brady *et al.* 1999). A recent study of terminally ill cancer patients (McCain *et al.* 2003) suggests that spiritual well-being offers some protection against end-of-life despair when death is imminent.

Spirituality may not always be protective, however. Those who cannot find meaning in their illness, or who are angry with God, may experience significant spiritual distress. Although this topic has received little attention from researchers, there is some evidence that tackling spiritual questions may raise troubling existential or religious issues. Patients may have serious doubts about their religious behaviour and whether or not it has been carried out in the correct fashion. In one qualitative study on prayer, about one third of cancer patients expressed concerns about the efficacy of their prayers. These concerns caused inner conflict and mild distress (Taylor *et al.* 1999).

What it is about being religious or spiritual which enhances coping is an interesting question. A number of factors are potentially of significance: the perception of God's support; deferring responsibility for illness and its outcome onto an omnipotent God; the cathartic effect of rituals and prayer and the social support provided by a religious community. There is evidence that higher levels of belief about God's control are related to higher levels of self-esteem (Jenkins and Pargament 1988). This issue requires further empirical investigation.

Coping with life-threatening illness in specific religious groups

All religions have difficulty answering questions about health and suffering. Perhaps the most common question asked is 'Why did this have to happen to me?' Often there is no answer to this question; in fact, it is not so much a question as an expression of emotional and spiritual pain. Religious people may seek some reason, often related to some wrongdoing, sin or failing of character. Others, although they do not feel that they are being punished, feel that the illness is somehow part of God's plan for them and they pray to discern this higher purpose. This higher purpose may be to bring about changes in themselves (such as acceptance or humility), or to deepen their spirituality, which in turn may facilitate coping. Even those who are not religious may feel a sense of guilt about their illness derived from the strong influence of Judeo-Christian tradition in Western culture.

Further issues of a religious nature often arise in those diagnosed with cancer. If God has caused the illness, the question arises whether one should seek a medical cure. Is it necessary to live through suffering? Does suffering have a redemptive or educational purpose? Overcoming suffering is often seen as a religious opportunity to demonstrate the mastery of the spirit over the flesh. All religions have to answer the question as to why God, who is seen as all compassionate and merciful and omniscient, does not prevent suffering. How can one interpret the apparent incompatibility between God's absolute goodness and the suffering of the innocent?

Case study: dealing with serious illness in Islam

In Islam sickness can be expiation for sin, an opportunity that God bestows upon those he loves. The Qur'an (67.1, 2) teaches:

> Blessed is He in Whose hand is the Sovereignty, and He is Able to do all things. Who has created life and death that He may try you, which of you is best in conduct, and he is the mighty, the Forgiving.

In Islam the purpose of life relates to many tests which must be undergone during life on earth. If these trials are passed, there will be eternal rewards. If they are failed, there may be punishments. The Islamic philosopher Rumi, in the *Discourses of Rumi* (FIHI Ma discourse 68, Arberry 1994), says:

> Those who are healthy do not look for God and do not see Him, but as soon as pain afflicts them, they cry out Oh God, Oh God, calling out and surrendering to God.

Health is seen as a blessing, both good and bad. Sickness is sent as a trial. 'When God intends to do good to somebody, he afflicts him with trials' (Salith el Bukhari vol. 7: page 373, Hadith 548). This is a blessing in disguise. Rumi says that Allah created suffering and heartache so that a joyful heart might appear through the opposite. Hidden things become manifest and known to us only by means of their opposite. Everything is determined by Allah. If a sick person can still remain faithful to Allah through the course of his or her suffering, trials and tests of illness, and still not oppose his or her destiny, endured patiently, there will be many rewards and recompenses for them.

It is taught that the more severe the trial and hardship, the greater the reward:

> I visited the Prophet during his ailments and He was suffering from a high fever. I said, 'you have a high fever. Is it because you will have a double reward for it'? He said, 'yes for no Muslim is afflicted with any harm but the Allah will remove his sins as the leaves of a tree fall down'.
>
> (Sahih Bukhari vol. 7 book 70 No: 550)

Despite the fact that Islam teaches a theory of predestination, it is still the responsibility of human kind to seek out medical help, although Allah ultimately determines whether doctors can cure. It is believed that no sickness is given which cannot ultimately be cured by Allah. According to Islamic teachings, the Prophet asked his followers to seek treatment for all illnesses, hinting that illness and medicine are both Allah's creations. Allah is seen as being in control of the beginning and end of life and therefore Islam stresses the importance of not becoming angry with Allah for giving us illness. This is ultimately a positive thing. Whether one has health or illness, it is the best that could ever happen. Ultimately, Islam teaches that to be miserable and unhappy because of self-pity, or angry over something which you cannot control, is not only futile but a complete waste of time. One should put one's trust in Allah, rather than lead life in extreme misery and sorrow (see Box 4.3).

Box 4.3

Abdul, a 55-year-old Muslim man from Bangladesh, regularly attended his local mosque. He prayed five times a day and described himself as devout. He developed cancer of the bladder two years before his death. What was striking about Abdul was that he was very calm throughout his illness. He emphasized how Islam helped him cope with his illness. Ultimately everything that happened was for the best. He explained that it was ultimately fated as to what would happen to him and there was no point being angry. After all, it was Allah who determined what happened. Abdul died peacefully in a local hospice. His family recounted how this was the will of God and nothing could be done about it.

Understandings of sickness in Judaism

God is portrayed in the Bible as morally good and describes himself as compassionate and gracious, slow to anger, abounding in kindness and faithfulness, extending kindness to a thousandth generation, forgiving iniquity, transgression and sin (Exodus 34: 6–7) and is described many times in the Bible as a healer. Illness is listed as one of the punishments God inflicts for sin. The Torah promises that if we obey God's commandments he will prevent illness in the first place (Exodus 15: 26; Deuteronomy 7–15; Leviticus 26: 14–26; Deuteronomy 28: 22).

> if you listen to the voice of The Lord your God and do what is upright in his eyes . . . all the sickness which I have set upon Egypt I will not set upon you, for I the Lord am your healer.
>
> (Exodus 15)

The question frequently arises as to why God allows humans to suffer and be miserable at all, other than when they clearly deserve it? However, the fact remains that in our everyday experience, the innocent do become ill and this still begs an explanation, even if the explanation is that we, as mortal human beings, cannot understand God's ways (Job 38: 2–4). There are other views in Judaism. For instance, the Torah reflects on *Yissurin Shel Ahava* (sufferings of love) 'those whom he loves the Lord chastises' (Proverbs 3: 12). The suffering individual is offered an opportunity for spiritual growth by examining his or her deeds and repenting: 'Let us investigate our ways' (Lamentations 3: 40). For an excellent discussion of the topic see Bulka (1998).

The Torah gives permission for doctors to heal. In fact, there is a positive obligation for those who are able to do so to use their skills and resources to heal the sick. The individual Jew, when ill, has an obligation to seek medical care. To this extent, Jews may not live in a community without a physician. Not only should Jews pray for God's help in bringing healing, they must also take steps to prevent illness and must consult physicians and follow their advice to restore health when they fall ill.

Jewish tradition has always asserted a close interaction between mind, body, emotions and will. God does not judge the body and soul of a person separately, but rather as one. Given the strong emphasis on the integration of body and soul, it is not surprising that, in Jewish law, the community's obligations to support healing include not only medical help but psychological and social support as well. Social support is essential at times of illness and thus the obligation to visit the sick (*Bikur Holim*). It is claimed that in visiting the sick Jews imitate God. Visitors should attempt to make the patients' lives meaningful.

Christianity

The question of unjustified suffering is at the heart of Christianity, which holds that Jesus suffered and died for the sins of humanity. Christians have not infrequently spoken of specific misfortunes as a punishment for sin. However, discussion of sickness in Christianity is complicated by the fact that different Christian denominations differ in their views concerning the relationship between sickness and human activity. Numerous verses in Scripture substantiate the view that physical healing in mortal life is not guaranteed in the atonement and that it is not always God's will to heal. Paul spoke of 'a bodily illness' he had (Gal. 4: 13–15). He also suffered a 'thorn in the flesh' which God allowed him to retain (2 Cor. 12: 7–9). Many modern day theologians and Christian leaders do not see a direct relation between sin and individual suffering. The picture of sufferings of the righteous Job in the Book of Job has presented many problems for this theory. For Evangelical Christians, sickness is part of the physical world caused by the fall of Adam. Jesus has taken on our sins and our suffering and therefore having faith in Christ can lead to healing.

A second view, held predominantly by Catholics, is that suffering is a way that a loving God tests faith and fortitude. According to St Paul, Christians should rejoice in suffering on account of the fact that it produces endurance, hope and character (Romans 5: 3–5). Catholicism emphasizes the close relation between physical and spiritual sickness. One view is that the sickness of the physical body is the cure for the spiritual body. Sickness and suffering strengthen the spirit and are part of a process of perfection (Hebrews 2: 10).

Another view is that a person may suffer as a means of increasing merit. Traditional Christianity affirms that Jesus voluntarily accepted suffering and death. He chose the path of suffering and offers a model of suffering, voluntarily endured, although there is nothing in his life which needed atonement. Suffering brings redemption. This theme of sharing in the suffering of Christ derives from Orthodox and Catholic theology and spirituality. Suffering can be seen as offering opportunities for spiritual and moral growth and development.

However, despite the value of suffering, Christianity by no means rejects medical treatments. The use of medicine is justified since the medical profession makes use of remedies that divine providence has provided in the natural world. Not only is the use of medicine justified, but physical health is a positive value to be promoted. Hope should be placed not in doctors but in Jesus Christ. There are, however, exceptions. Christian Scientists generally reject the use of biomedicine. Jehovah's Witnesses do not permit the use of blood transfusion.

Unlike Judaism, the Christian church exercises a healing role in a variety of ways. There is recourse to personal and group prayer and the laying on of hands is a common practice. In many churches there are services for the anointing of the sick and for the blessing of holy oil with which the sick can be anointed. In public services of Christian communities, the sick are prayed for and a charismatic ministry of healing exists in many communities. Holy Communion is brought to the sick, prayer services are held at the bedside and hands laid on the sick for healing.

Religious belief may, at times, prohibit the use of biomedical treatment as the example in Box 4.4 demonstrates.

Summary

The area of the emotional response to cancer across cultures is largely under-researched. There is a need for detailed ethnographic and psychometric studies in this area, with the development of culturally sensitive measurement scales. In relation to treatments for cancer related distress, there has been no specific work looking at the effectiveness of psychological and pharmacological therapies cross-culturally with cancer patients.

Various forms of psychotherapy have been shown to be effective in alleviating cancer related distress. One type of therapy, Supportive-Expressive group therapy, has been shown to be effective in reducing distress and pain in diverse cultures including France, Canada, Australia, Hong Kong and China (Spiegel *et al.* 1999). Therapies need to take into account cultural factors related to cancer, including varying propensities to discuss cancer, attitudes to death and dying, varying conceptualizations of autonomy, different family structures and differences in social support. How different types of psychological treatments might incorporate cultural factors is an exciting area for future research.

Box 4.4

A 50-year-old African American Christian Scientist developed a large lump in her left breast. She finally visited a physician who diagnosed breast cancer. By the time she saw him her lump was fungating. The doctors advised that she have an urgent mastectomy. She refused all intervention, arguing that God would cure her. This is consistent with Christian Science beliefs, which are not in favour of medical intervention. She died a couple of months later.

Further reading

Chochinov, H. and Breitbart, W. (2000) *Handbook of Psychiatry in Palliative Medicine*. Oxford: Oxford University Press.

Dein, S. (2003) Psychiatric Liaison in palliative care, *Advances in Psychiatric Treatment*, 9(4): 241.

Koenig, H., McCullough, M., Larson, D. (2001) *Handbook of Religion and Health. The Link Between Religion and Health: Psychoneuroimmunology and the Faith Factor*. New York: Oxford University Press.

Koenig, H. (2002) *Spirituality in Patient Care: Why, How, When and What*. Radnor, PA: Templeton Foundation Press.

Culture, treatment and cancer

Treatment for ethnic minority patients with cancer, both in the USA and the UK, has been demonstrated to be poorer than that for the general population. In this chapter the possible reasons for this are discussed. This will be followed by an examination of the role of cultural factors in delays in help seeking for breast cancer in various ethnic groups and its implications for health education. The chapter ends with a discussion of the under-representation of ethnic minorities in clinical trials and quality of life in these groups.

Poverty, race and survival

According to the US Census Bureau, in 2002 there were 285 million Americans, of whom 35 million (12 per cent) were poor and 44 million (15 per cent) were uninsured. A disproportionate percentage of African Americans (24 per cent) and Hispanics/Latinos (22 per cent) live below the poverty line compared to 8 per cent of White Americans who are poor. Proctor and Dalaker (2002) note that 25 per cent of the poor are found within 12 per cent of the population which is African American. While nearly 8 per cent of White people were considered to be in fair or poor health in 2000, nearly 13 per cent of Hispanic Latinos, nearly 14 per cent of African Americans and more than 17 per cent of Native Americans were in fair or poor health. Hence, levels of poverty clearly relate to levels of health.

Freeman (2004: 72–7) discusses the disparities in rates, treatments and survival of cancer in the USA. He points out how, since the mid-1970s, some progress has been made in understanding the causes of cancer, especially at the molecular level, and there has been a growth of 'effective' cancer therapies. There has been a decline in people who smoke cigarettes, which is significant, considering that tobacco is a cause of more than one third of cancer deaths. Related to this, there has been an overall decline in cancer mortality. The effects of these advances have been unequally distributed in different ethnic groups. For all cancer sites combined, residents of poorer counties of California have higher cancer death rates than residents in more affluent counties. Even when poverty rates are taken into account, some racial groups, e.g. African Americans and American Indians/Alaskan natives have a *lower* five year survival rate than non-Hispanic Whites. Within each ethnic/racial group, those living in a poorer county have the lowest survival rates.

This discrepancy in cancer mortality rates is by no means a new phenomenon. Henschke *et al.* (1973) reported an alarming increase in cancer deaths among African Americans in the preceding 25 years. A 'Special' Report on Cancer in the Economically Disadvantaged (American Cancer Society 1986) concluded that socio-economic disadvantage was responsible for poorer cancer outcomes in African Americans compared with White Americans and that poor Americans, irrespective of race, had a 10–15 per cent lower survival rate.

Another report in 1989 by the American Cancer Society (*Cancer in the Poor. A Report to the Nation*) pointed out that:

1   Poor people who lack access to quality healthcare are more likely than others to die of cancer.
2   Poor people endure greater pain and suffering from cancer than most Americans.
3   Poor people face major obstacles to obtaining and using health insurance and fail to seek needed care if they cannot pay for it.
4   Poor people and their families must make extraordinary personal sacrifices to obtain and pay for healthcare.
5   Cancer education and outreach efforts are insensitive and irrelevant to many poor people.
6   Fatalism about cancer prevails among the poor and prevents them from gaining quality healthcare.

The failure of biological theories to explain discrepancies in cancer survival across racial and ethnic groups

There is good evidence that, stage for stage, the survival of Black and White patients differs after a diagnosis of cancer. There may be a number of possible reasons for this: differing cancer biology; later stage at presentation of ethnic minority patients; differential treatments; and the higher occurrence of other coincidental illnesses in minority patients. Few studies have examined the proposition that this survival disparity might result from higher levels of coincidental and life-threatening diseases such as hypertension and poorly controlled diabetes mellitus. Bach *et al.* (2002) point out that a theory that cancer biology is different in Blacks and Whites has gained prominence, in reaction to the observation that Blacks have poorer survival than Whites, even when diagnosed with cancer of a similar severity. Following a review of 891 citations examining survival rates, these authors concluded that only modest cancer specific survival differences were evident for Blacks and Whites comparably for similar stage cancer. Therefore, differences in cancer biology within different racial groups are unlikely to be responsible for a substantial proportion of the survival discrepancy. Rather, it may be that differences in the stage of presentation and timing and quality of treatment may explain the different mortality rates (Bach *et al.* 2002). Another potential explanation relates to the differential racial response to various treatment modalities. This remains a relatively unexplored area. To date, there is little evidence that racial and ethnic groups differ in their response to specific treatments on account of biological factors (Shavers and Brown 2002).

However, biological theories purporting to explain disparities in cancer incidence and mortality between different ethnic groups cannot be completely ignored. Breast cancer provides an example of the complex relations between race/ethnicity, genetic factors, cancer risk and prognosis. The Surveillance Epidemiology and End Results (SEER) study (Li *et al.* 2003) of 95,523 patients with breast cancer over 50 years of age, found that women from ethnic minorities have a greater risk of oestrogen receptor/progesterone-receptor-negative breast cancer and that their tumours showed different histological profiles, compared with those of non-Hispanic White women. The authors note that these findings could partly explain the poorer survival among these populations. There is an emerging literature pointing to the impact of race and ethnicity on molecular pathways in human cancer (see Wiencke 2004). This point will not be discussed further, apart from stating that a comprehensive theory of race, ethnicity and cancer will need to take into account these biological factors.

Social suffering

Kleinman (1997) uses the term 'social suffering' to refer to what is done to and by people through their involvement with processes of political, economic, and institutional power. There are disparities in health on account of unequal privilege and power in racially and ethnically stratified societies. These differences in privilege and power significantly impact upon the treatments for cancer. He points out how 20 per cent of the world's population live in extreme poverty, with inadequate shelter, diet and security, which 'hack away' at the physical and mental health of these people. Although, in this book, we are not generally speaking of groups who live in abject poverty, the same processes of lack of power and privilege affect these people, a process which Kleinman refers to as 'everyday violence'. For him 'local power relationships refract the force of economic and political pressure so that some people are protected while others are more routinely and thoroughly exposed to the social violences that everywhere organise everyday life' (Kleinman 1998: 365). He makes the essential point that suffering must be understood at the same time both as individual and as collective. Kleinman's argument essentially is that individual suffering can only be understood in its wider social perspective and must take account of the ways in which different groups perceive and interact with the world. These interactions, in turn, are influenced by local and global power relations.

The effect of poverty

McCord and Freeman (1990) found that an African American man in Harlem had less chance of survival at the age of 65 than a male in Bangladesh. Cancer was the number two cause of death in Harlem. Two reports were issued by the Institute of Medicine relating to cancer disparities: *The Unequal Burden of Cancer* (Institute of Medicine 1999) and *Unequal Treatment: Confronting Racial and Ethnic Disparities in Healthcare* (Institute of Medicine 2003). Both reports documented the respectively disproportionate cancer burden in African Americans and the fact that African Americans, even at the same economic and health insurance status, were the least likely to receive the most curative treatment for cancer. They point out the need to understand the circumstances in which cancer occurs.

These reports cite poverty (low economic status), cultural injustice and social injustice as the three principal determinants of cancer disparities. Poverty is believed to drive health inequalities, more than other factors, by its influence on living standards and associated lack of resources, knowledge and information. It significantly diminishes access to healthcare and promotes risky behaviour including smoking and alcohol abuse. Members of ethnic minority groups are more likely to lack health insurance (Mills and Bhandari 2003). Those lacking insurance are more likely to present with later stages of disease and to die of their cancer. Ward *et al.* (2004) report that residents who live in counties that have greater than 20 per cent poor people have a 13 per cent higher death rate in men and a 3 per cent higher death rate in women. They are more likely to be treated for cancer at a later stage of the disease and are more likely to die from cancer.

Poverty acts through the prism of culture, which may augment or diminish poverty's expected negative effects. Cultural beliefs are related in some part to survival. For instance, Margolis (2003) reported that 61 per cent of African

Americans and 30 per cent of White Americans surveyed believed that lung cancer tumours might spread when exposed to air. This belief significantly influenced attitudes to surgical treatment. Nineteen per cent of African Americans and 10 per cent of White people opposed surgery based on this belief. Below, the specific socio-political factors related to survival are discussed.

Lack of health insurance

In 2002 20.2 per cent of African Americans and 32.4 per cent of Hispanics and Latinos were uninsured, compared to 11.7 per cent of the White population (Mills and Bhandari 2003). By 2050 nearly half of the US population will be comprised of minority groups. More than any other factor, whether a person has health coverage determines how soon that person will receive healthcare and whether he or she gets the best care available. Those who are under-insured or uninsured are less likely to receive appropriate healthcare. However, research has established that even when minority patients are insured at levels comparable to White patients, they receive a lower quality of healthcare for the same health conditions (Bach *et al.* 1999; Institute of Medicine 2003). African Americans and Hispanics tend to receive lower quality healthcare than White people across a range of diseases (including cancer, cardiovascular disease, HIV, diabetes, mental health and other chronic diseases). African Americans are also more likely to receive less desirable treatment, such as amputation of all or part of the limb, compared to White patients who are more likely to receive conservative surgery.

Lack of facilities

Areas inhabited by large numbers of minorities can pose barriers to care. Racial and ethnic minorities are more likely than White people to live in medically under-served communities and have fewer choices with regard to where they seek care (McCord and Freeman 1990). Twenty-eight per cent of African Americans and 30 per cent of Hispanics report having little or no choice in where to seek care, while only 16 per cent of White people report this difficulty. In the United States 'managed care' may pose a greater barrier to care for minority patients. For instance, one study found that African Americans were nearly one and a half times more likely than White people to be denied authorization for care after an emergency department visit for the same severity of problems (Lowe *et al.* 2001).

Stereotyping

Because of pressures to cut costs by spending less time with each patient, even well intentioned providers may resort to generalizations of stereotypes about patients who are members of racial and ethnic minority groups. There is good evidence suggesting healthcare providers, diagnostic and treatment decisions, as well as their feelings about patients, are sometimes unfairly influenced by patients' race or ethnicity. For example, research has found doctors rated Black patients as less intelligent and less educated, more likely to abuse drugs and alcohol, more likely to fail to comply with medical advice, more likely to lack social support and less likely to participate in cardiac rehabilitation programmes than White patients (Van Ryn and Burke 2000). This is even after patients' income, education and personality characteristics were taken into account.

Racism

Personal or historical experiences of racism, discrimination or violence might influence trust in health professionals and detract from help seeking. Those who perceive medical services to be discriminatory may well avoid their use and this might in practice worsen their prognoses. Racism might not be overt but institutional. The latter term refers to the collective failure of an organization to provide an appropriate and professional service to people because of their colour, culture or ethnic origin. This can be seen or detected in processes, attitudes and behaviour that amount to discrimination through unwitting prejudice, ignorance, thoughtlessness and racial stereo-typing, which disadvantages many ethnic people. This institutional racism may affect the minority patients' access to healthcare and the quality of care received. For instance, hospitals in the USA might adopt and implement policies that restrict admission. Ethnic minorities in the USA have higher unemployment rates compared to the general population. In the USA access to health insurance is often tied to employment. Those without jobs, or who are in low wage jobs, lack health insurance and therefore fail to obtain high quality medical care.

Communication barriers

Even if providers did dedicate an appropriate amount of time to patient care, communication can be a problem. Many minorities in the USA experience difficulties with English. Almost 12,000,000 people live in 'linguistically isolated' households (in which no one over 14 speaks English very well). Minority patients may have a difficult time finding healthcare providers who share their cultural and linguistic background. African Americans, Hispanics and American Indians are under-represented among healthcare professionals. As a consequence, one fifth of Spanish speaking Latinos recently reported not seeking treatment due to language barriers. Because of difficulty with communication, minorities demonstrate lower patient satisfaction with care, lower rates of appropriate follow-up, lower access to speciality care and poorer adherence to treatment plans.

There is also evidence that mistrust of healthcare providers might result in delays, as could the stigma associated with seeking care for some problems, such as HIV and AIDS.

Disparities in healthcare for cancer among ethnic minorities in the UK

There is little information in the UK about access to cancer treatments directly relating to ethnicity. There have been no comprehensive studies of access to cancer services for minority ethnic groups. A National Survey of NHS patients in the UK (Airey *et al.* 2002) tentatively suggests some disadvantage for minority patients. However, these findings are based on small numbers of ethnic minority patients, mainly living in London. For example, Black and South Asian patients were nearly twice as likely to report that their appointment for their first cancer treatment was postponed or cancelled than were White patients. These groups reported waiting longer after seeing their GPs before seeing a hospital doctor for diagnosis. South Asian patients were more likely than other groups to feel that they were not always treated with respect and dignity by hospital staff compared to other groups.

Other findings support the contention that British ethnic minority groups receive poorer cancer care than their majority counterparts. First, the proportion of people in the UK from diverse ethnic communities is lower than expected in trials of cancer treatments. This may result from sampling rather than access. Second, the proportion of people from diverse ethnic communities referred to specialist palliative care services is lower than expected. This is discussed in Chapter 7. Certain treatments may be problematic for ethnic minorities. For instance, donors for bone marrow transplants must be of similar ethnicity. Also, cultural and religious reasons may play a role in the lower donor rates to the bone marrow register, especially from South Asian communities. However, lack of access may be a key factor.

The use of traditional treatments

There is some evidence that when people move to a new country, although they may adapt to new ways and customs, they may return to their 'traditional' ways of thinking in critical situations. Such might be the case when diagnosed with cancer. For instance, those who derive from cultures with pluralistic medical systems such as India, where there is widespread use of Ayurvedic medicine, may find Western medical practices alien, despite growing familiarity with them (Ramakrishna and Weiss 1992). They may resort to Ayurvedic treatment for cancer, despite the lack of proven efficacy in this disease. This might be done at the expense of deploying Western treatments and potentially worsen their prognoses. The implication is not that Ayurvedic medicine has no effect on cancer, just that the case remains unproven. Similarly, although traditional Native American healers hold that cancer is a White person's disease and therefore Western medicine is appropriate, urban Native American breast cancer patients may refuse to participate in treatment until they participate in traditional healing ceremonies, which may require several months of preparation and might delay biomedical treatments (Burhansstipanov 2000).

Racism and disadvantage as physiological stressors

How these processes of poverty, disadvantage and covert or overt racism might impact upon levels of stress and in turn lead to pathology is only partially understood. There are close connections between the central nervous system and the immune system via hormones and immune mediators such as cytokines. There is emerging evidence that socio-economic status, stress and other culturally determined characteristics may directly impact on health and disease through the influence of the hypothalamic-pituitary-adrenocortical (HPA) axis and the sympathetic nervous system. The relation between neurological and immunological functioning is, however, complex and our understanding of the mediating processes is incomplete (Dein 2003). The term 'allostatic load' refers to the physiological and psychological costs of chronic exposure to fluctuating or heightened neuroimmune or neuroendocrine responses. The allostatic load is affected by environmental processes such as poverty. It is possible that these physiological changes in turn might enhance susceptibility to cancer or reduce cancer survival (Eskandari and Sternberg 2002; McEwen and Wingfield 2003).

Treatment and survival in specific cancers in the USA

Prostate cancer

Ethnicity may predict recurrence rates in specific types of cancer. For example, ethnicity has been examined as an independent predictor of recurrence after prostatectomy for prostate cancer (Grossfield *et al.* 2002). These authors found that Black ethnicity appeared to be an independent predictor of disease recurrence, after adjusting for pre-treatment measures of disease extent in patients undergoing radical prostatectomy. It was found to be particularly important in those with high risk disease characteristics. However, Black ethnicity, education and income were highly correlated variables, suggesting that sociodemographic factors may contribute to the poorer outcome in Black patients.

The contemporary attitude towards the treatment of early prostate cancer remains controversial. Some urologists argue for watchful waiting – just observing the patient and giving no active treatment. Shavers *et al.* (2004) examined whether race and ethnicity influenced watchful waiting for the initial management of prostate cancer. The authors found a higher proportionate amount of watchful waiting among African Americans and Hispanics compared to White patients. Urological surgeons were more likely to just 'watch and wait' in African Americans and Hispanics than in White patients. Whether this difference in attitude influences the eventual outcome of prostate cancer remains unknown.

Lung cancer

Bach *et al.* (1999) have examined racial differences in the treatment of early stage of lung cancer. The study found that there was a lower survival rate among Black patients with early stage non-small cell lung cancer compared to White patients. The authors explain the difference by the lower rate of surgical treatment among Black patients. Efforts to increase the rate of surgical treatment for Black patients appeared to be a promising way of improving survival in this group.

Breast cancer

Ethnic minority women in the USA may be more likely to present with advanced cancers (Polednak 1986; Long 1993; Li *et al.* 2003). Li, Malone and Daling (2003) looked at differences in breast cancer stage and treatment survival by race and ethnicity. This study looked at 124,934 women having primary invasive breast carcinoma between 1992 and 1998 and included 97,999 non-Hispanic White people, 10,560 Black people, 322 American Indians, 8834 Asians and Pacific Islanders and 7219 Hispanic White people. The study found that, relative to non-Hispanic White people, Black people, American Indians, Hispanic White people, Indian Pakistanis, Mexicans, South Central Americans and Puerto Ricans had 1.4–3.6 fold greater risks presenting with stage 4 breast cancer. Black people, Mexicans and Puerto Ricans were also 20–50 per cent more likely to receive or elect a first course of surgical and radiation treatment, not meeting the 2000 National

Comprehensive Cancer Network Standards. In addition, Black people and American Indians, Hawaiians, Vietnamese, Mexicans, South and Central Americans and Puerto Ricans had significantly greater risk of mortality after breast cancer diagnosis. American Indian and Alaskan natives have the poorest survival from all cancers combined, in comparison with all other racial and ethnic groups.

The study concluded that differences in breast cancer stage, treatments and mortality rates are influenced by race and ethnicity. The authors speculate that socio-economic factors are largely responsible for these differences. Disparities in treatment for breast cancer may indeed be related to socio-economic factors. Between 1988 and 1998, women with stage 1 and 2 breast cancer were less likely to be treated with breast conserving surgery and radiation if they resided in poorer, compared with more affluent, areas (Singh *et al.* 2003).

In terms of other cancers and their treatments, there has been relatively little research conducted in relation to ethnicity. African American women with cervical cancer were more likely in one study to go unstaged or go without treatment compared to White women (Merrill *et al.* 2000). Similarly for colorectal cancer, White people have been found to be more likely than other ethnic groups to receive aggressive treatments and follow-up after initially potentially curative treatment (Shavers and Brown 2002).

Hence, in the USA, there is substantial evidence that ethnicity and its socio-economic correlates significantly determine cancer prognosis in specific types of cancer. The complex associations between cancer, ethnicity, SES awaits further investigation.

Breast cancer in the UK

Velikova *et al.* (2004) examined tumour stage, diagnosis, treatment, patient and provider delays to diagnosis and treatment and survival of South Asian patients with breast cancer in Yorkshire, in comparison with the general population. This was a retrospective study, using the Yorkshire cancer registry population-based data on breast cancer.

The study found that South Asian patients were significantly younger at the time of diagnosis and presented with larger primary tumours. They received very similar treatment to the White British patients, but a higher mastectomy rate was noticed. Survival rate for Asian patients, after controlling for age differences, was similar to non-South Asian patients. South Asian patients had significantly longer patient-related delay between the initial symptoms and the presentation to GP and a slightly longer provider-related delay in terms of diagnosis and treatment.

The study concluded that the outcomes of breast cancer treatment were similar in South Asian compared to non-Asian patients. Asian patients, however, presented later to their GPs with larger primary tumours and more frequently had mastectomy.

There is some evidence in the UK that socio-economic deprivation may be associated with delay in presentation with breast cancer. Adams *et al.* (2004) examined whether women living in deprived areas of the UK were more likely to have advanced stage breast cancer at the time of diagnosis. The authors reviewed 12,793 women with breast cancer from the Northern and Yorkshire cancer register and information service. They found 13 per cent had advanced cancer stage at diagnosis and 31 per cent had high-grade cancer. These trends were stronger in women potentially exposed to breast cancer screening programmes. The study found strong socio-economic trends in the chance of both advanced stage and high grade of breast cancer at diagnosis. Women of lower SES were more likely to present with advanced stage breast cancer. The authors report that the results may have been confounded by the variations in use of hormone replacement therapy. These socio-economic gradients in disease progression at diagnosis may be due, in part, to socio-economic gradients in the uptake of breast cancer screening (Sutton *et al.* 1994).

To what extent do cultural beliefs and practices result in delay in help seeking for breast cancer in various ethnic groups?

Uskul (2001) has presented a good overview of the cultural factors relating to help seeking for breast cancer in Canada. The discussion here builds on his overview of the area. Early detection of breast cancer results in a better prognosis and reduced mortality (Foster and Costanza 1984; Machiavelli *et al.* 1989; Facione *et al.* 1997). In terms of help seeking, there may be significant delays between symptom development, diagnosis and treatment, which might derive from three sources. The first delay occurs between the recognition of the symptoms and the medical consultation. The second delay occurs from the time of consultation until the final cancer diagnosis. The third delay occurs from the time of diagnosis until treatment is initiated. Some women may experience significant help seeking delays. In about 20–30 per cent of women, the interval between finding breast cancer symptoms and seeking medical care is at least 2–3 months (Coates *et al.* 1992; Lauver and Ho 1993).

The existing literature relating to this delay in help seeking has predominantly focused on personal, demographic and psychosocial factors (Anderson and Cacioppo 1995; Burgess *et al.* 1998; Ramirez *et al.* 1999) with little attention being given to socio-cultural factors. There is good evidence suggesting that a delay in help seeking for breast cancer symptoms is more prevalent among some minority cultural groups than among Anglo Saxon women. Being a member of an ethnic minority group can result in late presentations of cancer (Vernon *et al.* 1992; Dibble *et al.* 1997; Bottorff *et al.* 1998). For instance, Black women tend to present with more advanced breast cancer when detected and consequently have poorer survival than White women once the cancer is detected (Bain *et al.* 1986; Polednak 1986; Long 1993). There is, therefore, a need to understand the possible reasons for this delay, in order that further interventions can be planned. This involves taking into account womens' conceptualizations of the causes, consequences and preventive behaviour in relation to breast cancer. These conceptualizations may vary across cultures. When ethnic groups migrate they generally hold onto some of their 'cultural baggage' even if they acculturate. Culture specific beliefs often re-emerge under threat of illness (Mo 1992).

South Asian women, delay and breast cancer

Breast cancer is becoming a major concern for many South Asian women, although there is some evidence that these women may underestimate the risk of developing breast cancer. A British study, examining beliefs among South Asian women about breast cancer, indicated that these women did not perceive themselves to be at significant risk of breast cancer and that they believed that breast self-examination was not necessary. Modesty caused them to be reluctant to allow male physicians to examine their breasts and they therefore preferred to consult female doctors about such problems (Bhakta *et al.* 1995).

A study of breast cancer detection practices of South Asian women in Canada, using a descriptive exploratory design (Choudhry *et al.* 1998), found that knowledge about breast cancer was generally low and that fatalistic beliefs were common. Only 5 per cent of the sample 57 South Asian women believed that cancer could be cured. Only half of the women had ever had a mammogram and only 21 per cent believed that detecting cancer early was important.

A Canadian qualitative study (Bottorff *et al.* 1998) examined South Asian womens' beliefs, attitudes and values in relation to breast health practices and the factors associated with engaging or not engaging in breast self-examination practices and medical help seeking. Four central themes emerged in explaining breast health related behaviour.

1 *Beliefs about a woman's calling:* Women believed that they had to keep the family honour, be modest and put others first. This modesty was taught to children early in their lives. South Asian Indian women considered showing the body to others as inappropriate. Women attempted to maintain the appearance that their family was healthy, that

their lineage was strong and that they were coping with their everyday lives.

2 *Beliefs about cancer:* Cancer was perceived as a latent killer that was incurable and caused much suffering of pain and fear. The disease was seen as part of one's destiny (*karma*) or God's will and therefore little could be done to change it. Treatment was considered worse than disease and in fact caused cancer to progress.

3 *Beliefs about taking care of the breasts:* Some women believed that they were not at risk from breast cancer. It was considered a 'White woman's disease' and therefore they were unlikely to get it. Many women felt uncomfortable about the idea of taking care of their breasts by touching them. Concern about symptoms was often shared with their family to seek their support, reassurance and comfort, although they would not talk about them with those outside the family. Women believed it was not wise to keep worries to one's self – that it was better to talk to someone than to keep bad feelings inside, which might, in fact, make health problems worse. Women were reluctant to seek medical advice without the permission of important family members. Doctors were generally trusted, however; unless a doctor told them to have breast screening, they would not think it was necessary.

4 *Beliefs about accessing services:* Women generally believed that it was important to be accompanied by family or a friend to medical appointments.

These attitudes affected women's confidence and competence related to breast health practices including breast self-examination, clinical breast examination, mammography, screening and help seeking in the case of any breast symptoms.

In another Canadian study Johnson *et al.* (1999) focused on South Asian womens' explanations for the causes of breast cancer. The study found that women believed breast cancer was caused by God's Will or divine power. This is consistent with the prevailing belief in *karma* or predestination – the belief that life is mapped out from birth and little can be done to change what happens. Women also believed that having cancer in the family increased their vulnerability. If cancer was present in the family, it was believed the women would have it, and conversely, if it wasn't in the family, one wouldn't have it. In both cases this belief led women to postpone or avoid help seeking.

Chinese women and help seeking for breast cancer

Research on Chinese women in relation to delays in help seeking for breast cancer have largely focused on their knowledge and beliefs in relation to breast cancer symptoms, perceptions of cancer curability, their participation in cancer screening, their health related practices, attitudes towards doctors and their views on women's roles in the family (Mo 1992; Facione *et al.* 2000). Mo (1992) in North America found most practitioners of Chinese traditional medicine or folk medicine held cancer to be incurable. In the National Cancer Institute (1981) 'Chinese-American Cancer Education Project' (quoted by Mo 1992) women held that cancer was difficult to diagnose and could remain undetected in the body forever and that the following caused the cancer: breathing polluted air; smoking and drinking; using aluminium and lead utensils; having certain chemicals sprayed on crops; frozen food; preserved food; noodles; raw food and salted fish. They expressed an overall sense of powerlessness in the face of the disease. Breast-feeding, eating soya products and high fat foods and limiting salty fish were held to be protective factors. Women generally perceived their risk of breast cancer to be low and several held that they were not vulnerable at all.

In Facione *et al.*'s (2000) study in North America, Chinese women conceptualized health in general as a precarious state that could be easily disrupted if one did not maintain a balance. Precautionary behaviours such as eating well, exercising, avoiding stress and performing virtuous deeds were deemed to be important in prevention. As a result of virtuosity and adherence to behavioural norms, women expected protection from serious illness. Modesty emerged as the principal reason why women were reluctant to be examined by male physicians. It is not surprising that 90 per cent of the gynaecologists in China are women, as there is less embarrassment in being examined by a female physician (Bhakta *et al.* 1995). First generation Chinese immigrants were more likely to make use of traditional Chinese medicine than Western medicine. The latter was considered over-aggressive and only used as a last resort. Chinese women mentioned they would only resort to physicians if traditional Chinese medicine failed.

Women mentioned their concern about the potential disruptive effect of breast cancer on their ability to care for their families. This is understandable in a culture where the needs of the collectivity are considered more important than the needs of the individual (Markus and Kitayama 1991). They are thus likely to avoid actions that would make them appear to be caring for themselves too much, which in turn might increase the burden on their family (Uskul 2001).

Black women, health seeking and breast cancer

A significant disparity in breast cancer survival between Black, especially African American, and White women has been widely reported (Gregorio *et al.* 1983; Long 1993). Black women have an approximately 20 per cent higher mortality rate for breast cancer in the USA compared with White women (Nemeek 1990); they tend to be diagnosed with breast cancer at younger ages and are likely to present with a more advanced stage of breast cancer than their White counterparts. There is evidence that Black women delay consultation with doctors more than White women (Gregorio *et al.* 1983).

People from socio-economically disadvantaged backgrounds lack access to health services because of diminished resources and non-availability of services (Neighbors 1987; Rice 1987). Even after controlling for socio-economic status, one still finds differences between Black and White women in terms of delay (Matthews *et al.* 1994). A number of factors above and beyond socio-economic deprivation may account for this delay: fatalistic attitudes, religious beliefs and the influence of folk beliefs about cancer.

High degrees of fatalism, a strong sense that men were not supportive of women's suffering, poor knowledge of breast cancer risk factors and the use of traditional healing emerged as themes in one study of 133 Black women in East Carolina in 1983. These themes were associated with advanced presentations of breast cancer. Matthews *et al.* (1994) analysed the narratives of 26 Black American women who presented with late stage breast tumours who were therefore assumed to have delayed a significant amount of time before seeking treatment for breast cancer. The narratives emphasized breast cancer as being ultimately fatal. It was seen as a supernatural disease, which was not subject to treatment with ordinary means, including medical ones. Another belief was that any discussion of the topic of cancer could make the cancer worse.

Long (1993), in a review of breast cancer in African American women, obtained similar findings to the above study. She also found that Black women did not adhere to the expected 'sick role behaviour', on account of their need to look after their families. They were more likely to assume responsibility for their condition and recovery, rather than seek and cooperate with experts.

Beliefs about Western medicine may influence the delay in help seeking. Snow (1983) examined the views of lower class Black women. These women felt that biomedical physicians did not understand their problem and were not able to effectively treat their illness compared to folk healers (Snow 1983). By contrast, there is some evidence that Black women prefer physicians to make decisions about treatment rather than deciding themselves (Gemson *et al.* 1988).

Greek and Greek Cypriots in the UK

Using a focus group methodology, Papadopoulos (2001) examined the attitudes of Greek and Greek Cypriots in the UK towards cancer. The findings suggested that cancer was generally feared and stigmatized in these groups.

All participants agreed that Greek and Greek Cypriot people did not like talking about cancer (in Greek, *kardinos*). The word 'cancer' was associated with bad things, sadness and fear. Participants held the disease to be caused by unhealthy lifestyles and stress. Some elderly informants held cancer to be caused by Satan.

Informants often found the messages about prevention to be confusing. Another general area of agreement was that many Greeks or Greek Cypriots died from cancer because they did not acknowledge any changes in their bodies giving them some early signs and therefore delayed going to the GP. Elderly women were embarrassed to talk about breast changes. Fear was the main barrier to seeking early help. Interestingly, there was a general agreement that cancer, if it was caught early, could be cured.

Hence, we can see that, in all the groups discussed above, cultural factors are significantly important in determining delays in seeking help with breast cancer. There are commonalities across these groups: similar notions of autonomy, the role of the family in decision making, the effect of illness on womens' functioning within the family, fatalistic attitudes to cancer and the importance of modesty in their relationships with physicians.

Health education programmes to minimize delays must be based on anthropological research

It is not solely problems of access to healthcare facilities, language barriers, economic conditions and lack of integration which are the major causes of delay in ethnic minority groups. Even if access is made easier, cultural factors may still prohibit the use of services. Health education programmes need to address fatalistic attitudes, issues of modesty and religious ideas. Messages may need to be targeted at the family rather than the individual. Knowledge of the health beliefs influencing delay is vital for the planning of interventions to target these beliefs and hence minimize delay. Health education programmes need to take into account perceptions of breast cancer as an illness, beliefs related to its causes and consequences, perception of Western medicines and physicians, sources of breast cancer information, level of perceived vulnerability and women's status in the community.

The first barrier to overcome is the linguistic problem. Reading material, radio and television programmes relating to breast cancer symptoms must be made more understandable, for example, by incorporating visual materials. Issues of poor communication between patients and physicians must be addressed and bilingual interpreters deployed where necessary.

Modesty emerges as an important factor in delay in health seeking. There is a need to address this issue and to incorporate more female physicians into the communities where this is an important issue. As mentioned above, some ethnic minority women prefer female physicians for gynaecological and breast related examinations.

Health education messages should be tailored according to the perceptions of cancer. This includes addressing fatalistic attitudes. If cancer is seen as a fearful disease, using fearful messages or using the word 'cancer' extensively can have a counter effect, rather than the effects aimed for. The word 'cancer' may evoke feelings of fear and helplessness and might inhibit help seeking. Incorporating fear appeals is common practice in health promotion campaigns. A recent meta-analysis (Witte and Allen 2000) synthesized the findings of more than 100 experiments testing the efficacy of fear appeals. The results indicated that strong fear appeals were more persuasive than weak appeals. However, if people become too frightened, they are likely to stop processing the message and the appeal may backfire. It is essential, therefore, that any message which incorporates a fear appeal (such as 'breast cancer is a major cause of death') also includes information to promote a high sense of efficacy in the recommended behaviour change.

In this analysis, messages that combined a strong fear appeal with a high efficacy message were found to be most effective. Fear provoking messages, used to motivate health seeking and preventive behaviour, are not likely to be effective with South Asian women and may intensify anxiety (Johnson et al. 1999). Positive messages, perhaps in the form of stories of successful cure, could be one strategy to motivate women to seek help. Stories, particularly of hope, successful detection and treatment, may be more effective (Bottorff et al. 1998).

In view of the fact that help seeking practices are strongly influenced by the family, health education must not be focused just on the individual, but on the total family. The fact that some ethnic minority groups hold their elders in high esteem signifies that they could play a major role in influencing womens' health practices.

The involvement of ethnic minorities in clinical trials

Ethnic minorities are under-represented in clinical trials and therefore denied the opportunity to examine the effects of ethnic factors on cancer treatments and their efficacy. Such representation could increase scientific knowledge about the health of ethnic minority groups and might be the basis for providing more equitable services for these groups (Corbie-Smith et al. 2004). Swanson and Bailar (2002) report on 261 randomized clinical cancer trials (205 focused on cancer treatment and 56 on cancer prevention). They were published in 11 scientific journals between 1990 and 2000. According to the review, more than 90 per cent reported age and gender but fewer than 30 per cent reported race and ethnicity. This study concluded that most cancer clinical trial reports failed to describe the race and ethnicity of participants.

The authors state: 'other studies have shown that the effect of the treatment and prevention effort does vary by race and ethnicity. It is imperative that we find ways to encourage minorities to participate in clinical trials to ensure they receive the benefits of these studies' (Swanson and Bailar 2002: 950).

When minorities are included in clinical trials, it does not seem that their participation is by design, instead it is by chance and it is unclear whether it is done to support the trial's initial hypothesis or whether it is done to generate a hypothesis. When the results are analysed according to ethnicity, differences in treatment and prevention outcomes are often found. Clinical trials do not include participants diverse enough to ensure broader applicability of results.

There is some recent research suggesting that ethnic minority groups are also under-represented in research studies including clinical trials in the UK. Mason *et al.* (2003) found that people of South Asian origin were under-represented in six clinical trials conducted by the Yorkshire Clinical Trials and Research Unit. There is some evidence that, with appropriate invest-ment in translators, participation in trials can be increased and ethnic minority patients can achieve representation in clinical trials (Cooper *et al.* 2003). Hence, there is a clear need to incorporate ethnic minority members in future clinical trials. How this might be done remains a challenging question.

Quality of life as well as quantity of life

It is not just the quantity of life, but also the quality of life, which is import-ant for patients with cancer. The term quality of life (QOL) is one now used commonly in the health services literature but is very difficult to define. The World Health Organisation (WHO) defines QOL as 'An individual's percep-tion of their position in life, in the context of the culture and value systems in which they live and in relation to their goals, expectations, standards and concerns' (WHOQOL Group 1993). This definition implies that cultural factors are important in QOL. What constitutes quality of life may differ according to cultural factors.

There is some controversy as to whether QOL is a suitable candidate for scientific measurement at all. There is, however, an emerging consensus regarding the domains making up QOL instruments. These generally include: physical health; mental health; social health and global perceptions of health and well-being. Kuyken *et al.* (1994: 5) argue:

> The way in which people define QOL appears to vary significantly across cultures (i.e. how people in a given setting define a 'good life'), as do the factors that affect QOL (i.e. access to and availability of healthcare, socio-economic conditions etc). Maintaining sensitivity to

this diversity, while producing cross-culturally comparable data, is a challenge currently facing QOL researchers working on cross cultural QOL assessment instruments.

To date, there have been no specific studies of QOL of cancer patients in the UK from different ethnic groups. On account of this we do not know whether or not there are differences in QOL between ethnic groups with cancer in the UK, or if the existing QOL instruments are broadly applicable. There is a larger body of work examining QOL issues among Black and ethnic minority groups in the USA. The findings of these studies are not necessarily transferable to the UK. There are a number of methodological problems in deploying QOL instruments derived from one culture in another culture. The vast majority of instruments have been designed using White middle-class respondents. Linguistic, cultural and economic differences may influence their cross-cultural validity. There may be a need to either adapt existing instruments or devise new instruments when working with different ethnic groups. The development of these culturally sensitive instruments might in turn provide information which can influence culturally specific treatments and supportive care and improve patient well-being. It is vital to include members of the culture being studied in the development of these instruments.

Studies of QOL in the USA among ethnic minorities suggest that spirituality is particularly important in the QOL of some groups, such as African Americans. The spiritual dimension is often not included in existing instruments. There have been some differences found in the USA between QOL in ethnic minorities and White Americans, however these differences might be attributable to socio-economic factors or levels of pain. African American cancer patients have been found to have similar QOL to the White majority, whereas Hispanics have been found to have lower QOL than the ethnic majority. For an excellent review of QOL in ethnic minority patients the reader is referred to Parker and Hopwood (2000).

Summary

This chapter has discussed the fact that ethnic minority patients, both in the USA and UK, receive poorer standards of treatment and have worse prognoses compared to the rest of the populations. Although access to appropriate healthcare is important in this respect, cultural factors may lead to delayed presentations, with consequent worsening of prognosis. Culture cannot be considered in isolation, but inter-relates with wider structural concerns, including deprivation and poverty. The provision of culturally informed health education is not in itself sufficient to remedy these disparities.

Their eradication involves major socio-economic changes. How this might occur is the subject matter of Chapter 8.

Further reading

Donovan, K., Sanson-Fisher, R. and Redman, S. (1989) Measuring quality of life in cancer patients, *Journal of Clinical Oncology*, 7: 959–68.
Smedley, B., Stith, A. and Nelson, A. (2002) *Unequal Treatment: Confronting Racial and Ethnic Disparities in Healthcare*. Washington, DC: National Academic Press.

6 Complementary and alternative therapies in oncology

Complementary and alternative medicine has been defined by Ernst *et al.* (1995: 506) as: 'The diagnosis, treatment and/or prevention which complements mainstream medicine by contributing to a common whole, by satisfying a demand not met by orthodoxy or by diversifying the conceptual frameworks of medicine'. It comprises a large and heterogeneous array of techniques utilized for both diagnostic and therapeutic purposes. Since the mid-1980s there has been a growth in the use of complementary and alternative medicines (CAM) for cancer patients both in the UK and the USA. In this chapter the possible reasons for the growth of CAM and their use in oncology are discussed.

The use of CAM in the USA and UK and reasons for its growth

In 1989 the *British Medical Journal* reported that about one in eight British people used complementary therapies, the most popular being herbal remedies, manipulation, homeopathy, acupuncture, hypnotherapy and spiritual healing. Middle-aged, middle-class women were the most predominant users of these therapies (Aldridge 1989). This number has significantly increased since 1990. A number of recent studies suggest that CAM are used by 25–50 per cent of the general population in industrialized countries (Eisenberg *et al.* 1993; Fisher and Ward 1994; Maclennan *et al.* 1996). A British telephone survey on the use of CAM found a one year prevalence of 20 per cent. Herbalism, aromatherapy, homeopathy, acupuncture, massage and reflexology were the most popular therapies (Ernst and White 2000).

Although the use of CAM generally appears to be common in both the UK and USA, there have been few studies which specifically examine its use in different ethnic groups. Lee *et al.* (2000) reported on the use of alternative therapies by women with breast cancer in four ethnic populations in the USA. The study used 30 minute telephone interviews with Latino, White, Black and Chinese patients. About half of the women had used at least one type of alternative therapy and one third had used two types. Most therapies were used for the duration of less than six months. The type of alternative therapy used, and the factors influencing the choice of therapy varied by ethnicity. Black women most often used spiritual healing, Chinese women herbal remedies and Latino women dietary therapies and spiritual healing. Among White women, 35 per cent used dietary methods and 21 per cent physical methods, such as massage and acupuncture.

In the United States the National Institute for Health, the nation's most prestigious research institution, has established an office of alternative medicine, now called the National Centre for Complementary and Alternative Medicine, which has a budget of over $100,000,000.00 and which has funded 10 university based centres for research on alternative and complementary medicine. Coulter and Willis (2004) argue that this is unlikely to be a passing fashion or craze. Many of the CAM group are embracing evidence based methods, with an emphasis on outcomes and the effect of the treatment compared with placebo groups.

The increasing use of complementary and alternative medicine within industrialized advanced Western nations is something of an enigma. As a social phenomenon it is not well understood or indeed much researched. It is interesting that the growth occurs in countries where Western science and scientific methods are generally accepted, as a major foundation for healthcare and 'evidence based' practice is a dominant paradigm. In Britain and the USA what appears to be happening is a social movement, featuring the increasing legitimacy of complementary and alternative medicine within the healthcare services. It is important, however, to point out that to a certain extent, people have always used CAM type treatments (in the past called home or folk remedies). What may have changed is the social acceptability of admitting to researchers or medical practitioners that they have been doing so. In developing countries most healthcare treatments, especially among larger, poorer sections of the population, have always been folk remedies or traditional healing, on account of the cost and lesser accessibility of conventional treatments.

Coulter and Willis (2004) suggest possible explanations for the rise in CAM use: the ageing population, the growing emphasis on chronic illness, and lifestyle related morbidity rather than acute illness. In such instances, where conventional medicine may be perceived to be less successful, the CAM may have much more to offer (e.g. the use of acupuncture for chronic pain).

The political climate and the consumerist ethic have fostered an attitude of individual enhancement and free and active choice, leading to self-assertiveness in healthcare as a reaction against the paternalism of bio-medicine. The most frequently cited reason for consumer use of CAM is dissatisfaction with conventional medicine's ability to treat chronic illness. There is some evidence to support this contention. Boon *et al.* (2003) explored the perceptions, feelings, ideas and experiences of Canadian patients with prostate cancer, regarding making decisions as to whether or not to use CAM. This study deployed focus groups and found that participants appeared more likely to be pushed towards CAM by negative experiences with the healthcare system than to be pulled towards CAM by perceptions about its safety or congruence with their beliefs about health and illness. Using qualitative interviews and a focus group, another study examined the experiences of eight women 'estranged' from biomedicine with a variety of cancers. Reasons cited by informants for abandoning conventional treatments and using CAM included anger concerning doctors' communication, taking control of their lives, belief in a cure, the provision of hope, mystical insights into healthcare and iatrogenic experiences of conventional treatments (Montbriand 1997).

However, the popularity of CAM has too often been dismissed as a sign of rejection of scientific authority and expression of new values of natural medicine, or of increased time and personal attention given by CAM practitioners. There are many reasons why people choose CAM; the choice cannot be explained solely by disenchantment with medicine or alternative ideology. A recent multivariate analysis failed to predict CAM use in relation to dissatisfaction with biomedicine in a national sample (Astin 1998). Sharma (1990) rightly points out that it is important to examine patient's sources of dissatisfaction with conventional medicine in some detail, since many of them do not relate straightforwardly to conventional medicine's failure to cure disease, as much as its failure to cure disease on terms acceptable to the patient. Many patients may be dissatisfied with their conventional treatments but do not use CAM. Factors apart from satisfaction, including the influence of advertisements and other family members, are likely to account for use of CAM.

The choice of practitioner may be influenced by a number of factors. A Canadian study examined the motivations of patients who chose to seek care from one of five different types of practitioners: family physicians; chiropractors; acupuncturists/traditional Chinese doctors; naturopaths and Reiki practitioners. The findings suggested that patients chose specific kinds of practitioners for particular problems and used a mixture of practitioners to treat specific complaints. The choice of type of practitioner is multi-dimensional (Kelner and Wellman 1997).

There may be other social trends mediating the use of CAM. A second explanation might be called the postmodern thesis (Coulter and Willis 2004). This suggests that social change (involving globalization) has accelerated. This has led to a decline in faith in the ability of science and technology (including medicine) to solve the problems of living (Crook *et al.* 1998; Siahpush 1998). There is some data suggesting that people who use complementary medicine are more likely to hold postmodern views (as opposed to scientific rationalism) and are supportive of individual perspectives, new age values (Astin 1998; Siahpush 1998) or are dissatisfied with the orthodox medical encounter. This includes a sense of not being valued sufficiently as a person within the medical system.

As Coulter and Willis (2004: 588) note 'Any explanation why more patients are choosing CAM must also take into account why patients are increasingly able to exercise this choice, have it met by CAM providers and, in some instances, have it paid for by the state and insurance plans'. There may be several broad social changes which are responsible for this. Of significance is the impact of the consumer movement on healthcare. A good example has been feminism, but it can also be seen in the gay movement, particularly around HIV, and the green movement. This returns control of health to the individual and control of the healthcare system to the community.

It is also significant that the growth of CAM has coincided, both in the USA and elsewhere, with the lessening of medical dominance. Coulter and Willis (2004) argue that for much of its history medicine has constrained CAM by ensuring that it was not taught in medical schools, that universities did not have research funding and did not get access to hospital laboratories or services that might have enhanced their services to their patients. It was also not covered by government insurance. Private educational institutions created by CAM providers did not receive funding. All these impeded significantly the legitimacy of CAM. The ideology was one of medicine claiming to be acting in the public interest. As the consumer movement gained in popularity and healthcare became politicized, this defence lost its legitimacy and consumers began to act in their own interests. There have been social trends towards individualism – which result in individuals being less prepared to accept traditional authority, including medical authority, and seeking greater levels of control and empowerment over their lives – a trend fuelled by the internet (Beck and Beck-Gernsheim 2002; Coulter and Willis 2004). The declining competitive advantage of conventional doctors, as bulk billing is abandoned, means that patients may be more willing to try alternatives, even though CAM is not cheap. As internet use grows, patients may find more and more useful information about CAM treatments, whatever the problems with some of this information might be.

Another related explanation for growth in CAM since the mid-1980s is increased migration and transmission of medical systems from other cultures. Treatments deriving from Eastern healing traditions (e.g. acupuncture, reflexology) are popular and highly marketed today and many people are travelling abroad to learn about these treatments. In a similar way, those trained in these types of treatments may migrate to the West. Certain premises of CAM enhance its appeal. Its perceived associations with nature, vitalism and spirituality might bridge the gap between the domain of medical science, emphasizing truth and strict causality and the domain of religion, with its moral freedom and self-chosen values (Kaptchuk and Eisenberg 1998). Related to this has been the growth of social green movements, with their preference for organic and non-chemical solutions to problems (Eastwood 2000).

The use of CAM in cancer

With the lay perception of cancer often being incurable and potentially fatal, it is likely that frequent resort is made to complementary and alternative therapies in this condition to ensure that all possibilities for cure have been tried. Attempts to 'cure' cancer and prolong life by complementary therapies have been widely reported in the media. The establishment of the ISSELS clinic in Germany in the 1970s and the subsequent claims that natural methods could cure cancer, attracted derision from medical professionals. In the early 1980s the Bristol cancer centre promoted the idea that diet, natural therapies, healing and other mind-body techniques could cure cancer. These ideas were not backed by sound empirical evidence finally leading to the Chivers report (1990), which suggested (although with little evidence) that these natural therapies were actually harming patients and that those using them were more likely to progress to an advanced stage of their cancer. Since the mid-1980s, claims have been made for the efficacy of a large number of CAM, ranging from dietary to homeopathic and herbal substances (e.g. laetrile and mistletoe), to psychological approaches such as visualization (Simonton et al. 1980; Spiegel et al. 1989), to acupuncture and various forms of massage such as reflexology and aromatherapy.

In the UK there is evidence that GPs are increasingly adopting a positive approach to complementary therapies, with more GPs themselves training in these therapies and using them with patients (Ernst 1995). The British Medical Association has recommended that doctors should be better informed about these treatments. However, there are medico-legal issues concerning their use including those relating to the training and qualifications of complementary practitioners. A similar situation exists in the nursing profession. There has been improved access within secondary care, with therapies such as acupuncture, homeopathy, massage and aromatherapy being offered for cancer in a number of hospital settings (Burke and Sikora 1993). In a survey of 190 hospices providing inpatient care in the UK (Lee and Whitehead 1998), 91 per cent of respondents provided some form of complementary therapies and those that did not were considering it for future development. It has been suggested that psychosocial care is provided at all stages of cancer and that there should be ready access to CAM (Calman and Hine 1995). However, the provision and access of support and complementary and self-help resources is extremely random and most support initiatives are led and run within the voluntary sector.

How frequently are CAM used in the cancer setting and why are they used?

There have been a number of studies of the prevalence of the use of CAM in cancer, the motivations for using them and how these relate to expectations of those with cancer. Surveys suggest that a sizeable proportion of cancer patients resort to CAM during the course of their disease (Ernst and Cassileth 1998; Grothey et al. 1998; Weis et al. 1998). Using computerized literature searches to locate all published studies documenting the prevalence of CAM among cancer patients, Ernst and Cassileth (1998) retrieved 26 surveys from 13 countries. The frequency of use of CAM in adult populations ranged from 7–64 per cent. The mean prevalence across all adult studies was 31.4 per cent. They comment on the fact that the variability was most likely due to the varying definitions of CAM.

In an overview of alternative therapies used by Canadian cancer patients, Montbriand (1994) found that physical alternative therapies alone were reported by 76 per cent of the 300 respondents. Studies of British women with breast cancer suggest that over a third of these women visit a complementary therapist at some time following diagnosis, with another 15 per cent using an over the counter product but not actually visiting a complementary therapist. Patients using CAM are more likely to be younger, of higher socio-economic status, more frequently female than the overall cancer population and are more likely to have used CAM prior to diagnosis with cancer (Downer et al. 1994; Coss et al. 1998; Crocetti et al. 1998). Of interest, in these studies the majority of women state that they would prefer the referral to come from a doctor. In another British study in the Hammersmith Hospital two thirds of cancer patients said that they would use complementary therapy if offered to them (Sikora 1997).

There has been some concern that patients with cancer will desert potentially curative conventional therapies in favour of unproven methods (Cassileth et al. 1991). In fact, patients with cancer rarely opt out of conventional therapy altogether (Cassileth et al. 1984). In most cases, alternative medicine is used as a complement rather than as a replacement for conventional therapy (Thomas et al. 1991).

In an American study 13 per cent of cancer patients receiving conventional treatments in a cancer centre were found to be using complementary therapies simultaneously including metabolic therapy, diet, megavitamins and spiritual/faith healing. Reasons cited included control of their disease, potential cure and the prevention or halt of metastatic growth (Cassileth *et al.* 1984). Cancer is a chronic disease for many patients and much of their distress and dissatisfaction results, not from the fact that cancer is incurable, but from the quality of interpersonal aspects of the care they receive. In one study of patients with breast cancer and Hodgkin's disease, those who perceived physician communication to be poor were more likely to use the Moerman diet than those patients who believed that communication was adequate (Pruyn *et al.* 1985).

There is some suggestion that many patients are prepared to use conventional treatments, even if there is only a small chance of cure (Slevin *et al.* 1990). This study reinforces the belief that for many cancer patients hope is the important issue. If hope is not imparted by conventional practitioners, some patients may seek it from complementary therapists. It is therefore important for doctors and nurses to provide a hopeful attitude when dealing with cancer patients.

Downer *et al.* (1994) studied 415 unselected British patients with cancer, over 18 years of age, using semi-structured interviews and postal questionnaires. She found that 16 per cent of the sample used complementary therapies including healing, relaxation, visualization, diet and homeopathy. Three quarters used two or more therapies. Therapies were used for anticipated tumour effects. There was generally high satisfaction with both conventional and complementary therapies.

Patients using complementary therapies were less satisfied with conventional treatments on account of their side effects and lack of hope of cure. Although patients cited anti-cancer hopes as their main motivation, the overall benefits obtained were psychological, such as the provision of hope and optimism. Unlike the situation in the USA, where metabolic therapies, diets and megavitamins predominate (Cassileth *et al.* 1984) in Downer's study, mind body therapies, healing and visualization were the most popular among the British group of cancer patients.

Is the use of CAM related to the stage of the illness? There is some evidence that resort to CAM is more common in those with more advanced disease. A study of women with breast cancer in Honolulu suggests that a greater prevalence of CAM use is associated with lower doctor satisfaction and greater severity of disease (Shumay *et al.* 2002). Similarly, in men with prostate cancer (Wilkinson *et al.* 2002), progressive disease was linked to more CAM use. Ninety per cent of men in this study held that CAM would help them live longer and improve their quality of life, while 47 per cent expected a cure.

There have been few studies which examine why cancer patients do *not* use CAM. A Canadian focus group study of 36 women with breast cancer (Boon *et al.* 1999) pointed to three main reasons why CAM was not used: cost, access and time. Although, in this study, families and friends generally supported the decision to use or not to use CAM, healthcare practitioners' reactions to CAM use were described as mixed. Not all patients who consider using CAM actually use them. Coss *et al.* (1998) interviewed 503 cancer patients attending a cancer centre in California and found that 16 per cent had considered using CAM for their cancer. However, only 6 per cent actually saw an alternative service provider. Although the use of alternative care is not high in this group, there is a fairly high awareness of CAM. Most had a familiarity with some form of CAM.

Patients were asked about the extent to which the traditional care they were receiving met their physical and psychological needs. Although most respondents reported that their physical needs were being met, only 30 per cent of the respondents felt that the need for someone to talk to was being met and 26 per cent felt that emotional support for themselves and their family were adequate. Two thirds of the patients agreed with the proposition that it would be good if treatment focused on the whole person, including emotional and spiritual needs. About half of the respondents believed that their doctor would be supportive of their interest in CAM, whereas one third felt their doctor would be critical. The study indicates the patient's desires to integrate mainstream medicine with CAM and suggests that patients use CAM in oncology for a number of reasons including a desire to be treated as a whole person, an intention to participate in a meaningful and active manner in their care, a sense that biomedicine does not address the spiritual and psychological needs of patients and an attempt to improve the quality of life rather than the mere prolongation of life.

Hence we may conclude that reasons for deploying CAM in oncology range from expectations about the effects of these treatments on tumour growth to purely anticipated psychological effects such as provision of hope and feeling that one is treated as a whole person. What is certain is that their use is fairly common and often plays a major role in a patient's overall treatment programme.

The question of efficacy

In terms of research, the question of efficacy (effect on disease progression, symptoms and psychosocial variables) has received most attention. The academic literature on CAM to date has been characterized by a number of methodological problems (Barraclough 2001). These include poor descriptions of techniques used, small and non-random samples and the gross over-representation of some therapies (e.g. herbs) compared to others (reflexology). Of the randomized controlled trials of cancer treatments, over half focus on herbs. There is little research on reflexology and aromatherapy, therapies which are commonly used in cancer care. The existing studies have been designed to answer questions which are of little relevance to clinical decision making. The research base in complementary medicine is extremely patchy, and there is an urgent need for a systematic appraisal of existing research. Databases such as CISCOM (an in-house data base of over 60,000 published papers organized by the Research Council for Complementary Medicine) and the Cochrane Collaboration complementary medicine field reveal that there have only been a small number of systematic reviews of complementary therapies and few of these are relevant to cancer care. Although many studies (including RCTs, cancer directed interventions, observational studies, phase 1 and phase II trials) had encouraging results, none showed definitively that CAM altered disease progression in patients with breast cancer. In fact, it is difficult to draw any conclusions from systematic reviews, apart from the fact that the studies are generally methodologically unsound (Seers and Carroll 1998).

There has been a call for CAM to be subject to the same rules of evidence assumed to be held for biomedicine. However, there are more radical positions arguing that it is only biomedicine that has empirical support and until CAM can demonstrate such support it should not be considered as a complementary alternative. This lack of evidence, however, seems to be having little impact on the growing use of CAM. Many providers of CAM are in fact convinced that their therapy defies the 'straightjacket' of reductionist research, arguing instead that it is individualized, holistic, intuitive, etc. and instead call for a 'paradigm shift' in research (Ernst 2000).

There is another response from the USA and the UK, which is to practise medicine in a way that selectively incorporates elements of complementary and alternative medicine into comprehensive treatment plans, alongside orthodox methods and diagnoses of treatment. This can be done in numerous ways, for instance, by doctors seeking training in CAM. The approach in the United States is exemplified by doctors learning acupuncture, homeopathy, Chinese medicine and Ayurvedic medicine. A second response is bringing CAM into traditional medical centres. For instance, osteopaths and chiropractors have been brought into primary care in the UK (Faass 2001).

Consumers may have a very different way of thinking to biomedical scientists. They may be less convinced by clinical trials and new drugs that have been deployed only to a well-defined group. In the eyes of the consumer, trying a herbal remedy that has been used for many centuries may not be an irrational step. CAM consumers accept the possibility of a different perspective or understanding of their illness and sometimes welcome it as it opens a window of opportunity for treatment. If consumers believe they are not getting broad enough advice or making adequate progress with conventional medicine, they may try an alternative approach, which can offer help. This is a pragmatic enterprise.

Does the CAM literature have negative psychological effects on cancer sufferers?

Can CAM use have negative psychological effects on patients? Stacey (1997) points out how much of the writing on cancer provides countless personal accounts of those who have successfully fought and survived cancer. The person with cancer becomes a hero through bravery, fortitude or fighting spirit. Cancer offers the sufferer the opportunity to reassess and re-evaluate their lives and to live it differently in the future. She points out how these accounts are very seductive. These narratives continue to pervade the cancer subcultures of contemporary Britain and inform many complementary and alternative approaches to treatment. According to Frank (1995), in the USA there has been a recent move away from these heroic narratives towards a different and less monolithic form of storytelling. This move has not yet significantly influenced the UK.

Although it is essential to foster hope, there is a negative side to all of this. Many of the books focusing on CAM actively cultivate the idea that it is possible to overcome cancer by willpower. For instance, in the popular self-help book *Heal Your Body: The Mental Causes For Physical Illness and the Metaphysical Way to Overcome Them*, Hay (1989) suggests that cancer can be overcome through mental processes. Apart from the fact that this assertion lacks scientific proof (Dein 2003), there is the possibility that sufferers from cancer might be made to feel guilty if their disease is worsening, as if they are not trying hard enough. Attention must be given to the messages portrayed by the alternative therapy movement such that patients are not made to feel guilty or despondent about their lack of improvement.

Summary

This chapter has examined social trends which mediate the rising use of CAM in the UK, USA and Canada. The growth of CAM and the decline of medical dominance are associated with broader cultural changes in society and its associated healthcare provision, along with the growth of the consumer movement that stresses increased choice and works to have these choices recognized as legitimate. CAM use is related to complex social and cultural factors including disillusionment with biomedicine and its increasingly technical approach, fragmentation of care due to specialization and the loss of bedside skills and changing conceptualizations of health in terms of balance, a return to the 'natural' and the importation of ideas from Eastern religions to the West. Another significant factor includes the fact that biomedicine has not proved successful against some lethal diseases such as cancer and many chronic conditions (Lerner 1984).

It appears that the use of CAM in cancer patients is fairly commonplace.

However, it is rarely employed as a replacement for orthodox medical care, but generally as an adjunct to it and is used as one of a range of treatment options. Many sufferers report significant positive benefits from their use, although it is important that patients are not given false expectations. There is a need to further assess their potential advantages and disadvantages in oncology.

Further reading

Barraclough, J. (2001) *Integrated Cancer Care: Holistic, Complementary, and Creative Approaches*. Oxford: Oxford University Press.

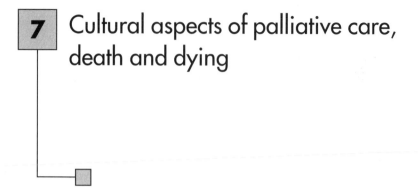

7 | Cultural aspects of palliative care, death and dying

Inequities in palliative care provision

The term palliative care refers to:

> An approach which improves quality of life of patients and their families facing life-threatening illness through prevention and relief of suffering by means of early identification and impeccable assessment and treatment of pain and other problems, physical, psychosocial and spiritual.
> (WHO 2002: http://www.who.int/cancer/palliative/definition/en/)

This chapter examines palliative care among ethnic minority patients, both in the UK and USA, particularly emphasizing inequities in provision of this care and the possible ways of addressing them. It then discusses anthropological approaches to death and dying and their implications for palliative care.

Inequities in palliative care provision

There is an emerging literature on the use of palliative care services by ethnic minority patients both in the UK and in the USA. This literature broadly points out two main themes. First, there is a marked variation in the quantity, quality and types of palliative care provided in different cultural groups. Second, there is some concern about the under-utilization of these services by minority and ethnic groups generally (Eve *et al.* 1997; Smaje and Field 1997; Hill and Penso 1995; Haroon-Iqbal *et al.* 1995; Karim *et al.* 2000; Haber 1999). Under-utilization might derive from the fact that these groups are not referred to palliative care services in the first place (related to the attitudes of health professionals), or the fact that the groups themselves do not wish to use these services (related to their own attitudes about end-of-life care).

The poor uptake of palliative care services can be explained in terms of three factors: need, demand and supply. Hill and Penso (1995) speculate that there may be several reasons for this poor uptake in the UK. The first three relate to decreased need among minority patients; the fourth relates to decreased demand in these groups:

1   a smaller proportion of older people in the minority ethnic population;
2   cancer not being the main cause of illness in Asian communities;
3   the incidence of cancer being lower among ethnic minorities than in the majority indigenous population;
4   little or no information about such services for minority ethnic patients and their carers, who might experience communication and language barriers.

However, there may be other reasons cited for this poor uptake: lack of awareness as to what can be offered; services not being culturally competent and the White Christian image of many hospices. In particular, different cultural groups might have varying patterns of dealing with advanced illness. There is a common assumption, often held by the ethnic majority, that ethnic groups 'look after their own' within extended families (Fountain 1999). This assumption may no longer be valid due to changing family structures and social and economic factors and some authors have seen this assertion as a stereotyped over-simplification (Atkin and Rollings 1996).

The use of palliative care services by ethnic minorities in the UK

The finding that ethnic minority patients under-use palliative care services is far from new. Rees (1986) reported on the use of palliative care services by immigrants in Birmingham, UK. He found their frequency of use to be much lower than that of British-born individuals. However, of those who were referred to the hospice, immigrants were more likely to receive hospice services compared to the majority population.

A qualitative study in the UK by Simmonds et al. (2001) aimed to identify formal and informal factors preventing or inhibiting access to hospice and palliative care services for ethnic minority patients. The study included South Asian people from Bangladesh, India and Pakistan. The findings of this study suggested that the obstacles to accessing hospice and palliative care services were often rooted in an interplay between formal processes and cultural barriers and assumptions.

Ethnic minority patients in this study were nearly three times less likely to have knowledge of hospice and palliative care services than ethnic majority groups. Most ethnic majority people learned about palliative care services through social interaction, word of mouth and informal sources. Ethnic minority groups were excluded socially from these kinds of information networks and disadvantaged from accessing formal sources of information through communication difficulties and lack of confidence. This was especially the case with ethnic minority women. The minority informants pointed out the desire to care for a sick or dying relative at home. This was deeply rooted in a sense of moral and religious duty in performing these roles and the honour (*Izzat*) of the family was closely bound up with these duties. However, the ethnic minority informants did point out that in the future these patterns might change as they became more westernized.

Racist attitudes have been cited as one reason for the poor uptake of palliative care services by ethnic minority patients. Firth (2001) reviewed research findings on improving access to palliative care for Black and ethnic minority groups in the UK. She summarized the main factors inhibiting access to palliative care services as follows:

> ... insensitivity, racism and lack of cultural awareness is still evident in the health service generally, including reports of racism, stereotypical thinking, ignorance and confusion on the part of the professionals. Racist patients have also challenged staff on the ward. Palliative care provision is based on existing western models of care.
>
> (Firth 2001: 4)

Ebrahim (1996) discusses the problems faced by ethnic minority communities, particularly ethnic elders, who do not make use of many statutory and voluntary services because they perceive these as being for the majority White population and insensitive to their needs. Heath beliefs emphasizing disease as God's will (for instance, in Islam) may explain why the process of rehabilitation is not widely understood by ethnic elders, who often possess a more fatalistic understanding of illness. Similarly, there is evidence that some ethnic minority groups do not disclose to the patient that they are dying and this might militate against accessing hospice care.

It is likely that minority ethnic groups would not favour hospice care because of isolation, poor communication, different food requirements and a desire to observe religious duties. Several studies (Hawthorne 1994; Gordon 1996; Karim *et al.* 2000) report linguistic and communication difficulties and cultural differences, different expectations of service provision, mistranslation of words by interpreters and the assumptions made by some GPs about the cultural appropriateness of hospital inpatient services for Black minority ethnic groups affecting referral decisions.

However, there is a need for good palliative care services for ethnic minority patients and their families, especially on account of the fact that the rates of cancer are increasing in these communities. As Karim *et al.* (2000: 476) point out in a recent study of the provision of palliative care services for ethnic minority patients and their families: 'people from Black/minority ethnic communities who are born in Britain may be reflecting the cancer patterns of the general UK population'. These authors go on to advocate that these groups therefore require appropriate cancer services. Similarly, a report by the Cancer Research Campaign (1996) concluded that people from minority ethnic groups in Britain were not getting the cancer care they needed. The findings suggest there are unmet needs for cancer care and there could be an increase in future needs, as minority populations adapt to westernized ways of life.

Improving access to palliative care services for ethnic minority patients

Hill and Penso (1995) recommend a number of strategies to promote ethnic and racial sensitivity in delivering palliative care services, as well as policies to improve access to and take up of services. The recommendations include: recording patients ethnicity; having an equal opportunity strategy; implementing a code of conduct stating explicitly what is and what is not acceptable behaviour by staff towards patients; ensuring ethnic staff recruitment and training; developing a communication plan; and ensuring culturally competent specific service provision.

One way of potentially making palliative care services more ethnically sensitive involves the provision of ethnic liaison officers. Jack *et al.* (2001) describe the role of the Macmillan Ethnic Minorities Liaison Officer (EMLO) in a Bradford Community Palliative Care Team. These authors postulate that this might enhance the uptake of palliative care services among these different minority cultural groups. The introduction of the pioneering role, Macmillan EMLO, in a palliative care context provides a unique opportunity to develop an understanding of the issues in this sensitive area.

The aim of the liaison worker is first to raise the profile of palliative care in the Asian community and with other agencies, such as social and voluntary services, and second to maintain and improve the quality of care provided to minority ethnic patients and their carers, by improving communication and facilitating their access to specialist palliative care services. They serve an important role, since communication problems often occur due to lack of fluency in English, especially among women and older people, with limited local availability of trained interpreters. The Macmillan EMLO in Bradford provides support with giving and receiving of information, religious and cultural matters, gender specific issues, benefits advice and bereavement support. Much of the work is carried out during visits with health professionals and followed up by subsequent visits and referrals are made to other service providers. EMLOs can advise on ethno-specific needs, such as housing and financial problems, which are common in ethnic minority patients (Spruyt 1999). Another aim is to promote the use of hospice inpatient and day patient services. The effectiveness of EMLOs remains to be evaluated.

Palliative care and ethnic minorities in the USA

There is a lower use of hospice care among minorities in the USA, including African Americans, Asian Americans and Hispanics / Latinos (Crawley et al. 2000; Ngo-Metzger et al. 2003; Greiner et al. 2003). A study in the USA (Harper 1995) concluded that hospice care is not accessed or utilized by minority groups proportional to their representation in the population as a whole (Harper 1995). Schumacher (2004) in *Hospice Care in the United States* notes that in 2002 only 9.2 per cent of hospice patients were African Americans, 4.3 per cent were Hispanic or Latinos, 8 per cent were Asian or Hawaiian Pacific Islanders and 3.7 per cent were classified as multi-racial or another race. In light of these findings, he strongly recommends that outreach and increased access for diverse populations is necessary.

Socio-political factors may be partially responsible for this refusal to use palliative care services. Crawley and La Vera (2002) point out that what is commonly experienced by many Black American patients is that medical care for minority patients and the elderly is different, and less optimal, than the care available for Whites. Crawley says, 'Herein lies the key to understanding the resistance on the part of some African Americans towards palliative care' (p. 775). As a group, Black people have been shown to prefer life saving interventions, even when such therapies could be deemed as physiologically and medically futile. She goes on to state that this preference evokes an image of 'going down fighting'. It may make sense to resist the notion of good death when prior access to basic preventive services was limited, in part due to institutional racism. Also, what may appear to those outside the community as unnecessary suffering during the dying process might be perceived within the community as an expected part of life's continual struggle.

The literature on health disparities in ethnic minority groups often identifies the notion of trust as an important influence on the attitudes and behaviours of African American patients towards palliative care (Crawley 2002). Social injustices may contribute to dispositional mistrust. Some physicians do indeed hold negative biases towards African Americans and this is reflected in their behaviour towards them. For African Americans, good palliative care needs to be part of a larger continuum of equitable care, which includes prevention practices and risk management, diagnosis and appropriate evidence based curative treatment. Efforts to increase utilization of hospice and other palliative care services will fail if they do not address the larger societal issues faced by minorities. Community based interventions and ones that have their origins within the community and therefore reflect these larger concerns, are more likely to be successful.

Preferences for end-of-life treatments among different ethnic groups

There may be cultural differences in preferences for end-of-life treatments. Terminally ill patients who are African American, American Indian, Hispanic Latino or British Caribbean may wish at all costs to prolong life and might rather pray for a miracle than accept hospice care (Reese and Ahern 1999; Koffman et al. 2003). Phipps et al. (2003) investigated the differences in attitudes, preference and behaviours regarding end-of-life issues in terminally ill patients and their designated family care givers. This study examined African American and White patients with end stage lung or colon cancer and their designated family care givers. Significantly more African American than White patients desired the use of life-sustaining measures, for instance, cardio pulmonary resuscitation or mechanical ventilation. Similar findings were reported by Blackhall et al. (1999). These findings may have significance for those looking after terminally ill ethnic minority groups who may have different preferences for treatment at the end of life. There is clearly a need for further research in this area.

The anthropological literature on death and ethnicity in modern societies

Field et al. (1997) note how the anthropological and sociological literature relating to death and ethnicity in modern societies is restricted in volume and scope. Most of this literature focuses on 'death beliefs' and funeral customs of different groups and discusses ways of dealing with the body and with the 'spirit' or 'soul' of the deceased. There is little said about the *experience* of death and dying in such groups. For example, in the UK there are accounts of Jewish (Katz 2000), Hindu (Firth 1996), and Sikh (Firth 1993b; Kalsi 1996) attitudes and practices related to death and dying. Deriving from anthropological rather than sociological backgrounds, these authors have generally focused upon 'cultural' descriptions of beliefs and disposal. They have ignored the process of change as minority ethnic groups adapt to new societies. There are some exceptions however. Jonker (1996) has addressed this issue among Muslim immigrants in Germany and highlights the central roles of religious leaders and undertakers who mediate between competing religious, cultural and practical demands.

The ritualization of death

How people think about death is culturally embedded. Culture provides a framework by which they can understand the process of death and dying and ultimately what happens afterwards. Each culture has its own unique approach to dealing with death, which may be more or less standardized, but almost always involves a core of understanding of spiritual belief, rituals and expectations. The existence of rituals relating to death is a fairly universal part of human experience. Although there are many definitions of the term 'ritual', a key characteristic is that they are a form of repetitive behaviour that does not have an overt technical effect. Rituals are usually public affairs which are symbolic, in that the behaviour or actions say something about the state of affairs, particularly about the conditions of those taking part in the ritual. In a Durkheimian sense, they express and renew basic values of the society. Rosenblatt (1997) points out that a ritual may be understood in many different ways. Essentially, the key to understanding a ritual seems to be what it defines. In terms of death and dying, they define the death, the cause of death, the dead person, the bereaved, the relationship between the bereaved, the meaning of life and major societal values.

The psychological effects of ritual

A number of authors have underscored the cathartic effect of ritual (e.g. Scheff 1979). Death rituals allow for the collective expression of emotion. Malinowski (1935), a prominent British anthropologist, argues that rituals occur to satisfy the psychological needs of the individual. In the case of death rituals, they facilitate the expression of grief. The funeral ritual is helpful and valuable for all who feel the loss of the deceased. It makes the loss real, it validates life and allows us to go on living. Attending the funeral allows us to deal with the loss, say goodbye, and reaffirms the importance of living. In modern Western cultures, rituals are kept in existence mainly for the sake of tradition. Their function is largely to 'heal' the living and to provide friends and relatives with some sense of closure, an opportunity to come to terms with the death and the opportunity to move on.

Types of rituals

Anthropologists have typically divided rituals up into three types: cosmic cycle or calendrical rituals (celebrating changes in the cosmic cycle); rituals of social transition (rites of passage); and rituals of misfortune. At times of misfortune, particularly illness, ritual may be deployed both as a form of diagnosis and as a form of treatment. In many societies sickness is presumed to be caused by a breach of a taboo and may be remedied by a ritualized offering to the gods, which might involve activities such as sacrifice. Rituals of social transition occur with pregnancy, birth, puberty, menarche, weddings, funerals and severe ill health, i.e. at major transitions in the life cycle. The rituals signify the transition of the individual from one status to another. When things lie in the no man's land 'betwixt and between', as the celebrated anthropologist Victor Turner (1969) calls it, they provide a sense of uneasiness, especially in those who prefer things more clearly defined. Individuals are vulnerable – in an abnormal position both to themselves and to others. Following physical death, the body is in an ambiguous state, often vulnerable to attack from outside forces or a direct risk to the living, hence the corpse must be protected and often those around the corpse must themselves be protected from pollution. Following the funeral, the person is incorporated into the world of the dead, or into the world of the ancestors, as is appropriate for the society which celebrates it.

Death rituals may involve isolation of the bereaved, the wearing of special mourning clothing or special markings and may require actions that seem to outsiders to be destructive or unpleasant, for instance, tearing one's clothing, not bathing or tearing one's skin. Ceremonies or rituals relating to death may be spread out over months or years. There is often a final funeral ceremony marking the end of mourning, the transition of the central mourners into new roles (for instance from wife to widow) and marking the transition of the deceased to a final stage. It may not be easy for a person who has emigrated to a secular community to carry out these rituals. A person from a society with elaborate death rituals, who is resident in Britain or the USA, may lack support for engaging in these 'necessary' death rituals.

In most non-Western societies, death is not a single event but a process whereby the deceased is transferred from the land of the living to the land of the dead. Hertz (1960) differentiates between social and biological death, between which there is a variable period of time. Social death is the end of the person's social identity. Social death normally occurs after biological death in a series of stages, including the funeral, mourning and annual rituals of remembrance. In some circumstances, however, a form of social death can be said to precede biological death often by many years. Individuals are still physically alive, but in a subtle way are less alive socially. For instance, the diagnosis of AIDS or cancer may have significant influence on how people react to the ill person leading to avoidance, and thus it represents a social death.

The rituals performed at death resemble those played out at other critical periods of the life of the individual. Van Gennep (1966) defines death as a rite of passage. According to him, all rites of passage follow a standard pattern. The rite of separation is followed by the rite of transition and succeeded by the rite of incorporation. The themes of separation, transition and incorporation mark every life cycle ceremony, although each is differentially emphasized according to the group and the occasion. Death ritual can be seen to contain several elements of separation, transition and incorporation. Symbolic of separation is the deposition of the corpse in the grave, coffin or crematory; burning the dead person's clothes, house and other possessions.

Mourning is transition. The mourners are segregated, both physically and socially. Normal social life is suspended for the mourners for a prescribed period of mourning and then activities are regulated by taboos. There may be reversal of normal social patterns during this liminal period. A good example is the Jewish *Shiva*, where for seven days beginning with the day of the funeral, the mourner is forbidden to leave home, to greet another person, to wear leather footgear, to bath, use make-up, shave or cut their hair or to have sexual relations. He or she sits on a low stool, or on a chair or sofa. From the 7th to the 13th day the person may not shave or wear new clothes. He or she must refrain from participation in festive activity for a full 12 months (Wigodor 1966). Following this transitional period the mourner returns to normal life.

Culture and mourning

Cultures vary in the ways that different kinds of deaths are dealt with. The meaning of the death, the rituals called for, the emotions felt, how the body is to be disposed of and one's ultimate relationship with the deceased, depend on factors such as whether the death is a suicide, drowning, the death of a child or woman's death versus a man's death, a violent death, etc. It is often the older generation who are more observant of the rituals and more dedicated to the cultural meanings and emotional forms that have been dominant in the culture. Cultures differ in who is allowed to grieve, who is the principal mourner and who is seen as experiencing the most loss within the given death. One cannot assume it is the widow or widower who has the most right to grieve. Eisenbruch (1984) describes some of the culturally patterned ways in which people leave a deceased among different social and cultural groups in the USA including urban Black people, Chinese, Italians, Greeks, Asians, Latinos and South East Asian refugees. Mourning customs vary. For instance, in the Irish wake, the dead person is watched by relatives for several days and nights. Sometimes there is feasting and drinking. Among Greek Cypriots there is a culturally patterned weeping and wailing, followed by a defined period of mourning, wearing black. The Jewish *shiva* has been briefly described above.

The management of death in modern Western contexts: from home to hospital

Processes of modernity, secularization, urbanization and social mobility result in a weakening of bonds with the ritual community which in previous times acted to protect against the experience of loss and buttress identity. The loss of religious interpretations of death and dying might lead to an increasing existential crisis and difficulty dealing with their effects.

A significant transition has occurred since the mid-1950s in the ways in which death and dying have been handled in Western contexts. Aries (1981), a prominent historian of death, points out how, until the middle of the twentieth century, death was a public process, people died in their homes and it was common practice for the body of the deceased to be 'laid out' at home. Death and dying were seen as natural parts of life and an integral part of existence. By the mid-1960s two thirds of all deaths occurred in hospitals and this figure has generally continued to increase since then (Addington-Hall 1993). There is some evidence suggesting that between 50 and 70 per cent of cancer patients in developed countries would prefer to be cared for at home for as long as possible and to die at home (Dunlop *et al.* 1989; Costantini *et al.* 1993). Whether or not the person actually dies at home, rather than in hospital, is dependent on a number of factors apart from their individual preference. One significant contributing factor is the level of social support at home (Ahlner-Elmquist *et al.* 2004).

Hockey (1990: 56) argues that the process of secularization has resulted in a transition from a religious to a medical framework in the management of death. The doctor, rather than religious professional, oversees the dying process. Other possible explanations for this transition include the development of medical, surgical and pharmacological technology which have occurred in hospital care and the changing family and occupational structures in the West, generally with increased involvement of women in the labour market and a consequent reduction in the availability of unpaid lay carers.

This process of hospitalization has had significant consequences. As Hockey (1990: 63) argues 'Given that traditional medical models are either preventive or curative, neither therefore addresses themselves directly to managing the implacable and incurable process of dying and bereavement.' Dying patients in hospital were often neglected, treated as non-persons for whom little could be done. The hospice movement can be seen as a reaction against this process of dehumanization and neglect of dying patients, emphasizing a more personal form of care in which the dying person, together with their family, are seen as the main unit of care and in which the dying person is responsible for making decisions about treatment. The influences of these social processes on ethnic minority patients and their carers remains to be studied.

Specific religious groups and palliative care

Religious and spiritual issues are often significant in those who are dying and spiritual care is an integral aspect of caring for those who are terminally ill. Cobb (2001) has provided a comprehensive overview of this area. Here the emphasis is upon specific religious groups which differ substantially from each other in their attitudes relating to death and dying and customs associated with them. The discussion below derives from Neuberger (1994). These 'ways of dying' are better conceptualized as ideal types and one cannot assume that every member of a specific religious group adheres to a similar belief system.

Judaism

Judaism is life affirming. In Jewish eschatology, ideas about the resurrection of the dead and the afterlife are vague. On account of the perceived sanctity of life, there are strict laws about not shortening a dying person's life, since it is considered to be something which is of immense value. It is, however, permissible to eliminate any external factor which is stopping someone dying. Jewish belief does not require a final rite while a person is dying. There is a brief *viddui* (confession), provided that the dying person is able to speak and wishes to recite it. But if the dying person does not speak the words of the *viddui*, or if a rabbi is not present, no Jew feels that the soul of the deceased is endangered in any way. Often, however, a dying Jew asks to see a Rabbi. In this way a person gets the chance of a private confession and the opportunity to say the first line of a prayer called the *Shema*: 'Here Oh Israel, the Lord our God, the Lord is one'.

Classical Jewish sources discuss several stages of the dying process, with legal and theological consequences attached to each. When first diagnosed with an irreversible terminal disease the person is a *terefah*: there is a deficiency in the person's organs that will eventually bring death. This category has important legal applications. In Jewish law, killing an incurably ill person is forbidden. However, one who does kill the person cannot be convicted of murder for it is to be presumed the victim's illness was part of the cause of his or her death. In the last moments of life, when one is like a flickering candle, one is the *goses*. Death follows – defined traditionally as the cessation of breath and heartbeat, but more recently as the absence of brainwave activity including the brain stem. In traditional Jewish teachings the soul does not abandon the body until three days after death. Jews have a variety of beliefs as to what happens to a person after that.

Following death the body is left for about eight minutes with a feather over the mouth and nostrils, which is watched for signs of breathing. If there are no such signs, the mouth and eyes are gently closed by the son or nearest relative. The arms are extended down the sides of the body, the lower jaw is bound up before rigor mortis sets in. Traditionally the body is then placed on the floor with the feet towards the door, covered with a sheet, a lighted candle placed just by the head. On the Sabbath, or Jewish festivals, the body cannot be moved. Following this initial limb straightening, the body must not be left alone. Orthodox Jews have a custom of enlisting watchers or *shomerim*, who stay with the body day and night reciting psalms all the time. This time is usually fairly short, since Jews are commanded to bury their dead as quickly as possible.

Post mortems are resisted by orthodox Jews and similarly the giving of organs for transplants is frowned upon generally. Following these formalities the funeral is arranged. For orthodox Jews, burial is the only option in a Jewish cemetery. For progressive Jews it may be possible to cremate them.

After the funeral, there is a formal period of mourning for seven days initially (*shiva*). Evening prayers are held in the home and relatives, friends and members of the community come to pay their respects. Many Jews find this a very comforting experience. It is often the last wish of a dying Jew that members of the family should say *Kaddish*, the mourner's prayer, for him or her. This can be a source of considerable comfort for a Jew.

Christianity

A belief in an afterlife is an essential tenet of Christian faith. At one extreme is a fairly fundamentalist view of Heaven and Hell. Those following Jesus's example will go to Heaven, a perfect existence. Those who disobey and do not follow Jesus's example will go to Hell, a place of torment. For many Christians, Heaven and Hell are concepts rather than statements of literal faith. However, unifying all the varying theologies is a view that a new spiritual birth takes place by accepting Jesus into one's life. For Christians, impending death is a time for looking towards the afterlife. They believe that Christians share the hope of a new life beyond death.

Beliefs about death and dying vary according to the different Christian denominations. In the Orthodox Church patients may request a bible, a crucifix and a prayer book. Some may bring in a small family icon, which can be quite valuable. Prior to death, the local orthodox priest may be asked to visit the patient. The priest will hear the last confession and anoint the patient with the oil of the sick and give communion. This is a significant event for Orthodox Christians. There are no restrictions about handling the body.

In the Catholic Church, in order to facilitate the process of dying, the family may bring along a rosary, medallions of the pope, saints or the Virgin Mary. The Virgin Mary is of great importance in Roman Catholicism; Catholics frequently pray through her and ask her for mediation. Occasionally, they may keep by their beds holy water from Lourdes or from other shrines thought to be places of miraculous cures. Following death and the 'sacrament of the sick', the family may ask for the patient's hands to be placed in the attitude of prayer, holding a crucifix or rosary. In the Protestant church the traditional Christian sacraments of baptism, confession, Holy Communion, laying on of hands and anointing are available if required. There are, however, fewer formally observed last rites than in Catholicism.

Islam

Certain elements of Islam are important for palliative care. The majority of Muslims are Sunnis and minority Shias. The practices around death vary greatly according to sects and subsects and are heavily influenced by culture. There is a great emphasis on modesty and it may be embarrassing for a Muslim to undress in front of medical and nursing staff. For men, nudity, even in the presence of other men, is considered offensive. Women will expect to remain fully clothed in hospital or in a hospice. This desire for modesty may cause considerable problems in these settings. They may react strongly to male doctors or nurses and feel humiliated by this experience. If possible, women should always be examined and treated by women doctors and men by male doctors.

A Muslim prays five times a day at set times: after dawn, at noon, mid-afternoon, just after sunset and at night. It is important to wash before prayer and stand on clean ground facing Mecca. Shoes have to be removed and heads covered. Terminally ill Muslims would want to carry on with washing associated with the ritual of daily prayers as long as possible, although technically the seriously ill are exempt. Washing in running water is important and Muslims wash their private parts after urination or defecation.

It is incumbent on all Muslims to fast during *Ramadan*. Many terminally ill Muslims feel strongly about *Ramadan* and wish to fast. The seriously ill are exempt from this commandment, however, those in poor health should fast a little if they can. Some terminally ill patients may decide to fast, not taking anything into their bodies by mouth, injection or suppository from dawn to sunset. Pain control may be rendered difficult if not impossible.

Muslims believe in the afterlife merely as one stage in God's overall plan for humanity. The death is God's will. It is wrong to struggle against this. Suffering and death are part of God's plan and it is one's duty to accept whatever God sends. Some very pious Muslims show no emotion at death, since it would suggest rebellion against God's will. However, grief can be displayed openly and crying and weeping are common.

While a Muslim is dying, families usually stay by the bed. The family perform the rites and ceremonies saying 'there is no God but God, and Muhammad is his prophet'. These are the last words a Muslim should say. If possible, the dying Muslim should lie with his face turned towards Mecca, while another Muslim whispers a prayer into his ear. There is no confession.

Following death, the body should not be touched by non-Muslims. The eyes should be closed, limbs straightened and the head turned towards the right shoulder. The body should be wrapped in a plain sheet, unwashed. The body is clothed in white cotton garments. Muslims are buried, never cremated. The burial takes place as soon as possible, usually within 24 hours. After the body is washed, passages from the *Qur'an* are read and the family pray. The body is taken to the mosque or graveside for prayers. In Islamic law the grave is unmarked, whereas in Britain it is the law that the body be buried in a coffin and that the grave is marked.

Mourning usually lasts for about a month and friends and relatives provide comfort for the bereaved. Mourners are brought food by relatives and friends. For 40 days the grave is visited on Friday and alms distributed to the poor. A widow should modify her behaviour for 120 days, staying indoors unless absolutely necessary, wearing plain clothes and no jewellery.

Hinduism

Within Hinduism there is great variability in how followers worship. Time is seen as circular, unlike the linear conceptualization of time in the West. Reincarnation, the process of life, death and rebirth, is a constant never-ending cycle. Hindus emphasize the philosophy of *karma*. What an individual does in this world affects what will happen to them in the next. His position in this life is dependent on his actions in the life before. A Hindu patient may well adhere to this philosophy and may be worried by the thought that this final illness is in some way his fault and may feel a sense of guilt. Some Hindus might regard their deaths as insignificant because of the certainty of being at one with God in the life after death.

Many British Hindus are influenced by Ayurvedic teachings, which advocate a regime of regular diet, sleep, defecation, cleanliness of the body and clothing, moderation in physical exercise and sexual indulgence. This forms the basis of Hindu medicine. Hinduism emphasizes purification, especially the purification of the body. They try to bath daily in running water, which renders one not just physically, but spiritually clean. Therefore, a dying patient might be keen to carry on this duty. Washing hands and rinsing the mouth before and after meals is essential and there is strict cleanliness in the handling and preparation of food. Beef is to be strictly avoided and many Hindus, particularly women, are vegetarians. Fasting is common among Hindu women, especially widows and elderly women. On the special festivals, men and women fast on regular days of the week.

There may also be problems with modesty. Hindu women may be reluctant to undress for examination and might be shocked at being given a bath by a male nurse and visa versa. There is reluctance to talk about genital, urinary and bowel areas. This may be significant in terms of painkillers and constipation.

Hindus require a time for meditation and prayer and this will continue in terminal illness. Being alone for meditation is of considerable importance among some Hindus. Images or pictures of God may be kept under the pillow or by the bed, as may prayer beads and blessings and amulets. Medical staff and nurses of Christian persuasion may be offended by the large pantheon of Gods in Hinduism. It is important not to question this, but to respect it.

Hindu priests are often called in to the dying patient and they may perform acts of worship or *puja*. They also help the dying patient accept death philosophically. A 'good' death is seen as a conscious decision on the part of the dying, who control both the conditions and the moment of death. Following death, some place the body on the floor and light lamps with incense burners. In all cases, cremation is the usual custom. After the death, there is a ceremony called *Streda*, whereby food offerings are brought to the *brahmin* who performs some rites for the dead. There is usually a time of isolation or segregation at this time, although the chief mourners go into retirement. Grief is expressed openly.

There is no restriction on non-Hindus handling the body providing it is wrapped in a plain sheet. Post-mortems are considered extremely objectionable and disrespectful to the dead.

Sikhism

The number of Sikhs in Britain is slowly increasing. Hindus and Sikhs are very similar in their doctrine of reincarnation, which affects attitudes to death. Each soul goes through repetitive cycles of birth and rebirth. Death is not a frightening thing, but the ultimate aim is for each soul to reach perfection and to be reunited with God, not having to come back into this world. Like Hindus, Sikhs believe in the doctrine of karma, the cycle of reward and punishment for all thoughts and deeds. The life in this world is determined by previous behaviours. This cycle could be altered by good and bad actions in previous lives. The Sikh's family normally remain with them while they are dying. They are responsible for all the last offices.

Following death, the eyes are closed and the arms straightened. The body is wrapped in a plain white sheet. Each Sikh is cremated wearing the five symbols of faith, *Kesh* – uncut hair; *Kangha* – a comb; *Kara* – the steel bangle; *Kirpan* – the symbolic dagger; and *Kaccha* – special underpants or shorts. Cremation occurs within 24 hours of death. The coffin will often go first to the family home and is open for people to pay their last respects. It then either goes to the Gurdwara or the crematorium directly where the service is held. The heir to the dead person, usually the eldest son will light the funeral pyre. The ashes are collected and usually taken to the Punjab and scattered there.

The whole family remains in mourning in the days following the death. Relatives and friends come and visit and bring comfort and support. Women wear white as a sign of mourning. After ten days or so, a special ceremony called *Baog* is held, which marks the end of official mourning. The complete reading of the *Guru Granth Shaib* occurs, either at home or at the Gurdwara. Then life goes back to normal.

Buddhism

There are a growing number of Buddhists in Britain, from a variety of different schools. Buddhism acknowledges that suffering and human existence are strongly linked. Although Buddhism emphasizes the importance of pain relief and suffering in general, a Buddhist who is dying does not want a clouded mind and therefore may not wish to take pain relieving drugs. It is important to have mindfulness, i.e. being aware of everything, and it is often difficult for nurses and doctors to deal with this attitude to pain. In fact, some Buddhists may refuse pain relief. The ultimate goal, in the Buddhist tradition, is to strive for acceptance of pain. Western clinicians may view this acceptance as the patient giving up hope, or resigning himself or herself to fate rather than fighting.

Through its doctrine of non-permanence, Buddhism fosters an acceptance of death. For these reasons, Buddhists may accept impending death easily and may look towards their next life with apparent equanimity. Buddhists are usually cremated after death. A ceremony is conducted by a Bhikku.

Summary

There is growing evidence suggesting a poor uptake of palliative care services by ethnic minority populations both in the UK and in the USA. There is a need for palliative care services to become more culturally sensitive. A special edition of the *Hospice Journal* (Infeld *et al.* 1995) notes that 'while many people are individually knowledgeable and culturally sensitive . . . few hospices have systematically planned services to culturally diverse groups'. Addressing inequalities in access entails more than a fact file approach involving teaching healthcare workers about the essential characteristics of different cultural groups (specifically aspects of death and dying for hospice staff). It involves making them aware of their own attitudes to racism and discrimination and the material conditions shaping the experiences of those from ethnic minority communities.

Further reading

Aries, P. (1981) *The Hour of Our Death*. London: Penguin.

Barley, N. (1995) *Dancing on the Grave: Encounters with Death*. London: Abacus.

Bloch, M. and Parry, J. (1982) *Death and the Regeneration of Life*. Cambridge: CUP.

Field, D., Hockey, J. and Small, N. (1997) *Death, Gender and Ethnicity*. London: Routledge.

Metcalf, P. and Huntington, R. (1991) *Celebrations of Death: The Anthropology of Mortuary Ritual*. Cambridge: Cambridge University Press.

Murray Parkes, C., Laungani, P. and Young, B. (1997) *Death and Bereavement across Cultures*. New York: Routledge.

Neuberger, J. (1994) *Caring for Dying People of Different Faiths*. London: Mosby.

8 Tackling inequalities in cancer outcomes

The preceding chapters have pointed out the gross disparities in cancer care for ethnic minority groups, both in the USA and the UK and this is reflected in their generally poorer prognoses compared to the general population. These disparities relate not simply to 'foreign health beliefs' and language barriers; a full understanding must take into account wider structural factors including poverty, deprivation and racism. Culture does not exist in a vacuum but articulates with wider structural concerns. As Freeman (2004: 76) notes 'Disparities in cancer are caused by the complex interplay of low economic class, culture, and social injustice with poverty playing the dominant role'. Poverty is associated with significant health risks such as increased use of tobacco, alcohol and obesity, which themselves increase rates of certain cancers. As discussed above, there is some evidence that racial/ethnic differences in behavioural risk factors do explain some of the racial/ethnic differences in cancer (McGinnis and Foege 1993; Colditz and Gortmaker 1995; Freeman 2004).

The solution to reducing disparities involves more than correcting belief systems; it must involve attention to overcoming these socio-economic factors, including poverty and racism. Eliminating cancer disparities will require sustained efforts on the part of governmental, private and non-profit organizations, as well as individuals engaged in cancer research, cancer prevention and cancer care (Ward *et al.* 2004). Potential solutions for addressing these issues may differ between different countries with different political systems, but I would argue that the principles are essentially similar across developed nations. This chapter discusses a number of initiatives for decreasing disparities in cancer care, ranging from national incentives to local health education strategies which focus upon individual risk factors and screening uptake. It emphasizes the role of cultural competence using data both from the UK and USA.

The multi-dimensional nature of addressing health disparities

Health disparities among minority patients have been attributed to a variety of factors: low socio-economic status; lack of access to quality health services; environmental hazards in homes and neighbourhoods; scarcity of effective prevention programmes tailored for the needs of specific communities; differential exposure to risk factors; and shortages of health professionals in urban areas where minority populations are high. These factors are exacerbated by perceived discrimination, poor communication between physician and patient (Vermeire *et al.* 2001) and lack of cultural sensitivity and cultural competence on the part of physicians and other healthcare workers (Rutledge 2001; Geiger 2001). Coleman-Miller (2000) points out that history can have a tremendous influence on creating barriers of mistrust towards physicians and hospitals for minority groups who have historically experienced racism. The legacy of the Tuskegee University experiment, in which Black patients with syphilis were used as guinea pigs, illustrates this well (see Jones 1993).

The culture of poverty is important as is the patient's ethnicity, social status and cultural background. Economic status might determine the ability of the patient to acquire medical supplies and other resources, such as running water, electricity, adequate space, healthy or specific diet needed for continuity of care and wellness. Decisions made about lower income patients' care must be sensitive to different degrees of access to resources.

Religious beliefs often influence the patient's decisions about medical treatment. On account of their religious faith, some patients may request diagnosis but not treatment, believing that God will heal them. It must be emphasized however that mainstream religious teachings actively encourage or even obligate the sick person to obtain help from biomedical professionals. If a treatment is absolutely necessary, healthcare providers might find it useful to consult and collaborate with the patient's spiritual leader to facilitate this treatment process. Those who seek mainstream medical care may also seek treatment from healers in their culture. Rather than discourage this, especially if the alternative treatment is not harmful, providers and their staff might want to incorporate traditional healing into the general treatment plan.

Traditional cultures place a greater emphasis on the role of the family and decisions about health treatments may be a family affair. Cultural communication may be enhanced by realizing that family integration is more important than individual rights in many cultures. It is important to determine who is the appropriate person to make decisions and clarify and discuss the important ethical disagreements with them.

Much of the American literature on access to healthcare focuses on access to health insurance. It is well reported that health insurance coverage is less in every major minority group than for White people. Strategies to increase access to health insurance are important and necessary to decrease disparities in access owing to economic reasons, but the means to decreasing cultural and linguistic barriers lies in the provision of culturally and linguistically sensitive services to increase understanding and improve quality of care.

What can be done about inequalities in health? The US situation

The US healthcare system has traditionally employed two opposing strategies for targeting minority health. In the first approach, race is downplayed or negated in health analysis. In the second, involving 'blaming the victim', the claim is made that minorities experience poor health on account of 'pathological' behaviour including making a choice to smoke, drink heavily, consume the 'wrong' foods, engage in unprotected sex and violent behaviour or to lead sedentary lifestyles. Cultural beliefs are perceived by the mainstream to be 'outdated', or worse, signs of ignorance.

Despite the improvement in overall health, the majority of the American burden of health disparity continues to disproportionately affect minority populations. In response to these disparities, a number of major initiatives to improve the health of minority populations have been implemented (DHHS 2001). The main focus for reductions in disparity is on six key areas, which affect racial and ethnic groups differently at all life stages: infant mortality, diabetes, cardiovascular disease, cancer screening and management, HIV/AIDS and child and adult immunizations (DHHS 2001).

The Institute of Medicine document *Unequal Treatment* (2003) argues for a comprehensive multi-level strategy to eliminate healthcare disparities and makes a number of recommendations to this effect. It is important to raise awareness, among health professionals and the general public, of the healthcare gap among healthcare providers, their patients and purchasers of care. Patients can benefit from culturally appropriate education programmes to improve their knowledge of how to gain access to care, and how to participate in clinical decision making. Healthcare professionals need to learn how to understand and manage the cultural and linguistic diversity of patients in the healthcare system. Cultural sensitivity training should be integrated early into the education of future healthcare providers.

Health system interventions must be based on published clinical guidelines. Barriers to care must be overcome by providing translators. It is important to ensure that the physicians' financial incentives do not overly burden or restrict minority patients' access to care. Healthcare access may be improved by the use of community health workers. It is important to monitor data on patients' access and utilization of healthcare services by race, ethnicity and primary language. Publicly funded health systems should improve the stability of patient provider relationships, by establishing guidelines for patient caseloads. The proportion of under-represented US racial and ethnic minorities should be increased among healthcare professionals, to improve access to care among minority patients. The US Department of Health and Human Services should encourage health plans and federal and state payers to collect, monitor and report patient case data by ethnic and racial group.

National incentives in the USA to eliminate cancer disparities

There are a number of initiatives occurring in the USA to eliminate cancer disparities. The Clinton administration instituted a number of ongoing initiatives, including the upgrading of the Office of Minority Health to a Centre of Minority Health and Health Disparities like the National Institute of Health. A centre is more influential in setting a policy and influencing budgetary expenditure and can award grants. The National Cancer Institute's office of Education is currently updating its material on pain and symptom management to make it more accessible and culturally appropriate. The American Cancer Society has prioritized, as one its main aims, the elimination of disparities in cancer outcomes. The Inter-cultural Cancer Council is bringing together organizations to collaborate around issues of minority health and disparities of outcomes.

In 1999 the US Department of Health and Human Services (DHHS) Office of Minority Health first proposed national standards for culturally and linguistically appropriate services (CLAS) as a means to correct inequalities that exist in the provision of healthcare. They address the need for all people entering the healthcare system to receive equitable and culturally sensitive healthcare and are primarily directed at healthcare organizations. These standards represent the first national standards for cultural competence in healthcare. The 14 standards are made up of guidelines and mandates for all recipients of federal funds (see Box 8.1). Following these guidelines, there have been many efforts across the country to develop formal and informal curricula for teaching cultural competence in health service settings. These efforts have been largely isolated, each institution and organization developing its own discreet curricula independently and up to this point, standardized curricula for cultural competence have not been developed.

Box 8.1

National standards for culturally and linguistically appropriate services (CLAS) include:

1 Healthcare organisations should ensure that patients and consumers receive from all staff members effective understanding and respectful care provided in a manner compatible with their cultural practices and preferred language.
2 Healthcare organisations should implement strategies to recruit, retain and promote at all levels of the organisation a diverse staff and leadership that are representative of the demographic characteristics of the service area.
3 Healthcare organisations should ensure that staff, at all levels and across all disciplines, receive ongoing education and training in culturally and linguistically sensitive service delivery.
4 Healthcare organisations must offer and provide language assistance services, including bilingual staff and interpreter services at no cost to each patient/consumer with limited English proficiency at all points of contact in a timely manner during all hours of operation.
5 Healthcare organisations must provide patient/consumers in their preferred language both verbal offers and written notices, informing them of their right to receive language assistant services.
6 Healthcare organisations must assure the competence of language assistance provided to limited English proficient patients/consumers by interpreters and bilingual staff. Family and friends should not be used to provide interpretation services (except on request by the patient/consumer).
7 Healthcare organisations must make available easily understood patient related materials and post signage in the languages of the commonly encountered groups and groups represented in the service area.
8 Healthcare organisations should develop, implement and promote a written strategic plan that outlines their goals, policies, operational plans and management accountability/oversight mechanisms to provide culturally and linguistically appropriate services.
9 Healthcare organisations should conduct initial and ongoing organisational self-assessments of CLAS related activities and are encouraged to integrate cultural and linguistic competence related measures into their internal audits, performance improvement programmes, patient satisfaction assessments, and outcomes-based evaluations.
10 Healthcare organisations should ensure that data on the individual patients/consumer's race, ethnicity and spoken written language are collected in health records, integrated into the organisation's management information systems, and periodically updated.

11 Healthcare organisations should maintain a current demographic, cultural and epidemiological profile of the community as well as a needs assessment to accurately plan for and implement services that respond to the cultural and linguistic characteristics of the service areas.

12 Healthcare organisations should develop participatory, collaborative partnerships with communities and utilise a variety of formal and informal mechanisms to facilitate community and patient/consumer involvement in designing and implementing CLAS related activities.

13 Healthcare organisations should ensure that conflict and grievance resolution processes are culturally and linguistically sensitive and capable of identifying, preventing and resolving cross-cultural conflicts or complaints by patients/consumers.

14 Healthcare organisations are encouraged to regularly make available to the public information about their progress and success for innovation to implement the CLAS standards and to provide public notice in their communities about the availability of this information.

(Source: Federal Register 65(247): 80865–80879)

These national initiatives reflect a recognition that culture and language are central to delivery of health services. The 14 standards mentioned in Box 8.1 are directed primarily at healthcare organizations and represent a comprehensive set of recommendations and mandates for implementing culturally and linguistically appropriate services at all levels of organization. Individual providers are encouraged to use the standards to make their practice more culturally and linguistically accessible (Federal Register 65(247): 80865–80879).

Addressing priorities in research

In 1997 the US Congress requested a review of the research programmes of the National Institutes of Health relevant to ethnic minority and medically underserved populations. In response to this, an Institute of Medicine Committee was set up in 1998 to review the status of cancer research in relation to these underserved groups. Several recommendations emerged from this review (see Haynes and Smedley 1999). The need to define clearly the 'special populations' which are underserved was underlined. The committee emphasized the need to include survival data for all ethnic groups as well as for medically underserved populations and the importance of expanding behavioural and epidemiological research to further elucidate the relationship between cancer and cancer risk factors associated with various ethnic minority and medically underserved groups. They pointed out the importance of moving away from 'race', based upon fundamental biological differences, to a greater appreciation of the range of cultural and behavioural attitudes, beliefs and lifestyle patterns that may affect cancer risk across these groups.

The committee called for the Office of Research on Minority Health to be more active in coordinating, planning and facilitating research relevant to ethnic minority and underserved populations. One significant recommendation was that more emphasis should be given to cancers that specifically affect these groups. In relation to researchers, the need to expand the number of ethnic minority investigators and include them in all advisory and programme review committees was given high priority.

A significant part of the document discussed the need to improve patient's understandings of research and consent procedures and to facilitate recruitment of minority and underserved groups into clinical trials. Issues such as mistrust, literacy and other issues that may pose barriers to the participation of such groups in research were highlighted.

Finally, the committee proposed a regular reporting mechanism, to increase NIH accountability to the US Congress and public constituencies.

The situation in the UK

Although there has been some attention paid to addressing health disparities in ethnic minority groups in the UK, this work is still at an early stage. A British study commissioned by the Department of Health (Alexander 1999) found that there was a lack of research on minority groups and, in fact, the NHS policies excluded minority participants from trials. Similarly, there was an under-representation of minority leaders in the NHS and Department of Health. The Department of Health acknowledges that it is 'working to mainstream these issues in everything we do as part of our programme of modernisation for specific priorities for action'. The Department of Health study found significant disparities in the care of Black Asian and other minority groups, including differences in disease prevalence and mortality rates, access to care, quality of services and delivery of services. These findings will be deployed to improve ethnic minority care and further examine disparities in health.

Improving ethnic minority healthcare locally in the UK through health education: lessons from primary care

The principles to be discussed below, although focusing on British primary care services, can be applied to healthcare systems including secondary care and healthcare in other parts of the world. There is evidence that British ethnic minority patients consult with their GPs at rates which are higher than or similar to those of the general population (Gill *et al.* 2003). These higher GP consultation rates may reflect greater ill health and social disadvantage. However, they may be due to other factors, including poor communication or poorer outcomes from consultations. Primary care services are often underdeveloped in inner city areas, and are often insensitive to different cultural needs. There is evidence that British ethnic minorities are not given adequate time, do not feel listened to, are not examined properly and given appropriate explanations and that they may experience negative attitudes and cultural insensitivity from professionals (Fassil 1996; Yee 1997). On account of language barriers and poor availability of interpreters, people may feel uninformed about different services and how to access them. Kai (2003: 27) provides several recommendations for making primary care services more culturally sensitive and appropriate:

1 *Patient profiling:* There is a need to better define the local populations in terms of ethnicity, religious beliefs and information on language groups. At present this data is not collected consistently and appropriately.

2 *Empowerment of reception staff:* Barriers to access may be reduced by employing staff who reflect cultural diversity. Reception staff should be sensitive to patients' gender preferences for health professionals. For instance Muslim women should be able to access female GPs for specific problems.

3 *Raised awareness of services and health issues:* There is the need for services to consider whether the information given to users is culturally sensitive. This includes leaflets, audiovisual displays and resources which are accurate, appropriate for local communities and translated into relevant languages. There should be collaboration with local community and voluntary organizations, press, radio, television and schools to raise awareness of health related issues.

4 *Appointment systems:* Appointments may need to be made longer for certain groups where interpreting is required. This may necessitate significant changes in current working patterns.

5 *Culturally sensitive care:* Services should be acceptable to all patients and should be sensitive to the cultural values and beliefs of people from British minority ethnic groups. There is a need to scrutinize health service provision in terms of the care provided, including the provision of health promotion and education programmes.

6 *Enhancing communication:* Attention should be paid to the verbal and non-verbal aspects of communication in ethnic minority groups. There is a need for some degree of linguistic proficiency in staff working with these patients, unless they involve interpreters in their care. Since language barriers are often a major obstacle to carers, especially women and older people from South Asian and Chinese populations, it may be

helpful to recruit staff from British minority ethnic groups. There may be a need to incorporate professionally trained interpreters into the work situation.

7 *Cultural sensitivity:* Professionals must acquire locally relevant cultural knowledge and understanding about beliefs, diet and religion. Each patient should be treated as an individual and individual needs and variations recognized.

8 *Health education and promotion must be made culturally appropriate:* Targeting and delivering health promotion must involve the views of local communities who play a seminal role in planning. Their reactions to proposed methods and settings and the effects of interventions, not only on the target health issue, but also the wider aspect of the community's life, must be assessed.

9 *Developing a diverse workforce:* Over 7 per cent of NHS staff are from British ethnic minority groups. Local healthcare workforces should reflect the ethnic diversity of local communities. Issues of discrimination and racism, which may reduce the numbers of British ethnic minority people seeking employment in health services must be addressed. There is a need to recruit nurses and professionals allied to medicine from minority groups.

10 *Working with communities:* Local communities and their expertise should be engaged in the planning of services. This includes voluntary groups and individuals whose views should be valued.

11 *Inequalities must be tackled and extra support should be provided to disadvantaged groups:* There is a need to target resources and support to disadvantaged areas of most need. For instance, practice premises may need to be improved or poor staff recruitment addressed.

12 *Ethnic diversity awareness must be increased:* There is a need to provide greater awareness of ethnic diversity in training programmes for health professionals.

Developing cultural competence: more than learning about ethnic differences

The topic of cultural competence is currently one of great interest in the area of health provision. This relates to the changing demographic structure in the USA and UK and the increase in proportion of ethnic minorities. Historically, healthcare providers have ignored the diversity of cultural beliefs and practices about illness, health and well-being. The previous chapters have looked at the ways in which individuals in each culture seek healthcare for cancer and determine medical needs. There is much anecdotal evidence which suggests that many healthcare providers have little knowledge about traditional health beliefs and practices. This is not to undermine the great efforts that have been made in many parts of the USA and UK to increase cultural sensitivity.

However, cultural competence is more than an awareness of the health beliefs of specific immigrant populations and effectively communicating with patients who do not speak English. The term cultural competence may be defined as a set of congruent behaviours, practices, attitudes and policies that come together in a system or agency, or among professionals, enabling effective work to be done in cross-cultural situations (Cross *et al.* 1989). As Kai (2003) points out, effective cross-cultural communication means being sensitive to an individual's culture in its broadest dynamic sense including ethnicity, socio-economic background, education and religion. It is more than adopting a factfile approach to learning. Health professionals themselves *must be aware of their own cultures* and how their cultural backgrounds influence interactions with patients.

Rather than understanding their attitudes towards cultural diversity, health professionals often prefer to learn about ethnic differences such as dietary or mourning practices in different ethnic groups (Kai *et al.* 2001a). Despite this they might still, consciously or unconsciously, hold stereotyped or racist attitudes toward minority groups and therefore continue to discriminate against them. As discussed above, racism is a pervasive feature of healthcare both in Britain and the USA and can range from direct to institutional racism, whereby the way in which services are provided invariably disadvantages some ethnic groups. Changing attitudes is not easy. However there may be two ways of addressing racism and prejudice: first, better training that can inform all staff throughout the health services, allow them to become aware of their own attitudes and prejudices and sensitize them to racism and stereotyping; and second, achieving clarity about expected responsibilities and standards of behaviour in practice. The British Race Relations Amendment Act (2000) sets a legal precedent for ensuring that these standards are followed. Clinical governance frameworks can articulate standards of non-discriminatory practice and behaviour, this behaviour can be audited in the future.

This facilitation of cultural competence is by no means a panacea. Bigby and Perez-Sable (2004) note how training in cultural competence has been touted as a means to decrease health disparities, although this assertion remains unproven. Cultural competence is a difficult construct to measure and there is little information about how it should differ across racial and ethnic groups (Pena *et al.* 2003).

The teaching of cultural competence to healthcare professionals

The process of cultural training must become embedded in the education, assessment and accreditation of health workers (Kai *et al.* 2001b). First, Kai emphasizes the need to develop greater awareness of attitudes to difference and behaviours relating to these attitudes. Second, he points out the importance of participating and promoting equality and diversity training and reviewing current working practices. There is still much to learn about which strategies will encourage this sort of reflexive practice. Cultural training in the UK has been either patchy or non-existent among health professionals. In the UK the subject of teaching about culture to health professionals has received some, albeit little, attention. Dogra (2001) evaluated the implementation of a cultural diversity module in the undergraduate programme using a questionnaire before and after the programme. Following this intervention, there was a significant increase in positive attitudes toward and knowledge of different cultures (Dogra 2001). However, there is no research specifically examining how this cultural knowledge translates into clinical skills or better outcomes. There is, however, some evidence that cultural diversity training is becoming more popular in British medical schools (Dogra *et al.* 2005).

The discussion and teaching of cultural competence is an emotional activity and approaching issues of diversity and difference may generate a lot of discomfort in health professionals. People may react to the term in a number of ways, ranging from deep anger and hostility or lack of interest, to a deep appreciation and interest in the issue. To a large extent this is due to the inability of most people to deal with issues of racism. In order to respect other people's cultural values and beliefs, it is important for culturally competent organizations to work collaboratively with communities to determine priorities, solutions and strategies.

Specific teaching about culture in American medical schools has been relatively rare until the 2000s. A study by Flores *et al.* (2000) found that only 8 per cent of US schools and no Canadian schools had formal courses on cultural issues. The study pointed out that only 35 per cent of US medical schools addressed the cultural issues of the largest minority groups in their respective states. The American Institute for Research put together a document entitled *Teaching Cultural Competence in Healthcare: A Review of Current Concepts, Politics and Practices* (March 2002), which points out the fact that training physicians to care for diverse populations is essential. Other studies support the notion that the provision of culturally competent services can potentially improve the health of minorities by improving physician-patient communication and delivering healthcare in the context of each patient's cultural beliefs (Vermeire *et al.* 2001).

US healthcare organizations are beginning to make reforms in their policies to better support cultural competence. In 2001 the Liaison Committee on Medical Education issued higher standards for curriculum material in cultural competence never before required in medical schools. Many professional organizations in different areas of health have instituted policies, initiatives and projects and have even developed training materials to promote cultural competence in healthcare.

Health promotion: empowering minorities and the use of community health educators

In the Ottawa Charter for health promotion (WHO 1986) the World Health Organisation called for health promotion through empowerment, advocacy, community participation and organizational change. In line with this, one contemporary model of health promotion in oncology is the community health educator (CHE) model for cancer screening services. The core principles of heath promotion are community participation and empowerment. Much health promotion activity still continues to encourage individuals to change their behaviour through information-giving alone. This may not be effective, partly because of differing models of autonomy and time which exist in some groups compared to the educated professionals who plan health education programmes. Disadvantaged minorities who live a precarious existence may live each day one at a time. Planning ahead (for instance changing diet to prevent cancer in the future) might be alien to a group of people and hence this 'middle class investment model' (involving planning for the future) may not be part of their cognitive repertoire.

Empowerment and community participation

Health promotion initiatives, which serve communities and not just individuals, are central to the new health promotion movement. There is a need to understand the social, political and economic determinants that affect people's health and health behaviours. This includes acknowledging inequalities in the health experiences of disadvantaged and vulnerable groups and the associated imbalances of power that exist between health professionals and members of these communities. Empowering these communities necessitates that health professionals share power with them, thus enabling them to set and achieve their own health agendas. They must be involved in defining community health agendas, but also in the planning and delivery of health promotion activity in their communities (Chiu 2003). This new health promotion practice involves two major aspects:

1 Identifying community needs: Those delivering health promotion programmes must involve communities in identifying their own health priorities and increasing awareness of the wider social determinants of health as perceived by local communities and health outcomes defined by the government. For instance, to prevent cancer requires communities to recognize that cancer is a significant health problem and to define for themselves the ways in which health related behaviours can be changed.
2 The involvement of communities in monitoring and evaluation: The definition of what constitutes an effective health outcome from a specific intervention must be decided by the community itself. Lessons learnt from past interventions should be deployed in planning future interventions as part of a regular 'learning cycle'.

The community health educator model

The community health educator model was developed through participation-action research in order to address the low uptake of cervical and breast cancer screening among minority ethnic women. Central to this model are community participation and empowerment (Chiu 2003). Lay members of local communities are recruited and trained to develop health promotion as CHEs. These CHEs involve users of screening services in the planning and delivery of health promotion programmes in three stages.

In the first stage, focus groups are run to identify health promotion needs. In the next stage, health interventions and training workshops are developed. In the last stage, these interventions are implemented and evaluated by involving community members and professionals in focus group interviews. There is a feedback cycle and future interventions can be planned from this.

Several potential benefits derive from involving local communities in health promotion initiatives, these include: improving the quality and acceptability of services, the development of more appropriate linguistically and culturally sensitive health promotion resources, such as photo stories, and the opportunity for a lasting relationship to be established between primary care practices and their communities (Chiu 2003).

Many health districts in the UK have adopted this CHE model to encourage uptake of cervical and breast screening among ethnic minority women. CHEs work closely with practice managers, practice nurses and receptionists to identify ethnic minority women who have not attended screening. The model awaits evaluation.

In return for providing local knowledge, health professionals need to share technical knowledge with CHEs so that they can translate technical and biomedical terms. CHEs require knowledge of cancer screening and must learn the attitudes and skills needed by effective community health educators and promoters. There is therefore an obligation on health professionals to ensure that CHEs are appropriately taught.

Summary

Both in the USA and in the UK, any improvement in the health status of ethnic minorities must flow from a strong research agenda. This kind of research must be population driven. There is a need to devise new paradigms for research and their assessment among minority groups. The community must be involved in this process and community members must be trained to collect data which is potentially more accurate than that obtained by outside researchers. They should be involved in the process of data analysis and interpretation. This type of research benefits both the minority and majority population, since health education flows in two directions rather than one.

Further reading

Haynes, M. and Smedley, B. (1999) *The Unequal Burden of Cancer*. National Academic Press.
Spector, R.E. (1996) *Cultural Diversity in Health and Illness*, 4th edn. Stamford, CT: Appleton & Lange.

9 Conclusion: an agenda for future research

This book has examined how cultural and ethnic factors influence the diagnosis, treatment, prognosis and reactions to cancer. Cancer must be understood as a biocultural disease which is cultural to its core. Anthropologists and other social scientists have a major role to play in cancer care in terms of research, teaching and facilitating culturally appropriate care for sufferers. The evidence presented in this book suggests a role for anthropological insights in cancer care. This might be achieved through running short courses for clinicians or through the development of masters and doctoral programmes (for instance an MSc in culture and oncology) in universities. From the clinical perspective there will be increasing need for health professionals to be trained in cultural sensitivity and to obtain cultural knowledge about the populations with whom they are working.

Although some would contend that anthropology is a theoretical discipline, I would argue that medical anthropologists should consider how their theoretical perspectives might be 'clinically applied' and brought into healthcare contexts. A number of publications have begun to address these issues. For example Hahn (1999) examines how anthropological ideas can be integrated into public health programmes including those related to cancer. Some medical anthropologists have expanded their horizons to look at 'macro' influences on health and the ways that political and economic factors influence health inequalities (Singer and Baer 1995). These ideas are seminal in addressing such inequalities. This impetus towards clinically applied anthropology is reflected in the increasing numbers of applied anthropology courses in universities in the UK and USA.

Paradoxically, some advocates of the critical anthropological approach have taken issue with clinically applied anthropology, arguing that it fails to take account of the inherent power and class differentials between patients and practitioners. A major exponent of this position is the physician anthropologist Michael Taussig (1980) who points out that by helping physicians to understand patients better, anthropologists who are directly involved in patient care are unwittingly perpetuating the existing class structure and exploitation. This position appears rather extreme. A knowledge of patients' backgrounds is of course essential to good patient care and one aim of clinically applied anthropology is to enhance this knowledge base among health professionals by introducing anthropological themes such as the notion of culture, ethnocentrism, eliciting patients' perspectives, the disease-illness distinction and the importance of understanding illness in an holistic context. The challenge for medical anthropologists is to translate their theories into practice, to develop what Christman and Johnson (1990) label as 'prescriptive theory'.

There are two potential dangers of clinically applied anthropology which merit discussion. First, although it is common and I would argue acceptable for anthropologists to advocate on behalf of the communities they represent, they should be aware of undermining the expertise of clinicians and must attempt to maintain positive relationships with health professionals. Second, in their interactions with these professionals, they need to emphasize that 'culture' is a flexible, dynamic construct inter-relating with racism and social class and move beyond the simplistic 'cookbook' or factfile approach to culture that has been criticized above. Only by doing this will they prevent the problems of cultural stereotyping which are still prevalent in health care contexts.

What might future research in 'anthropological oncology' focus upon? There are several areas of significant interest in this respect. First, more work is needed to examine how rates of cancer and cancer mortality differ according to ethnic groups. What risk factors are culturally related? How do different cultural groups in fact understand notions of risk and prevention? Better systems are required for recording ethnic data. Future epidemiological research requires more sophisticated notions of race and ethnicity and understandings as to how these concepts are related to wider socio-structural concerns, including socio-economic status, poverty, deprivation and racism.

Second, there is a need for work examining in greater detail how understandings of cancer are culturally variable and how groups explain this disease and their attitudes towards it, especially issues of stigma. It is only by understanding these factors that the heavy burden of cancer can be reduced. Beyond this, it is important to further understand how these attitudes and understandings (including issues of fatalism) influence help seeking and ultimate prognoses. How can fatalistic attitudes be addressed and changed and what are the implications for health education? A related area is the role of the family in prevention, medical decision making and health seeking and their influence on health communication. Ethical issues, such as disclosure and informed consent, require further examination. For instance there is a need for work examining how bad news might be communicated among minority groups in Europe and the USA and especially how these issues are dealt with when the predominant view of the ethnic majority is to disclose the diagnosis and prognosis of the illness. The wider area of cancer communication in general provides fertile ground for future research. How do patterns of communication relate to psychological outcomes in cancer? How do patterns of communication about serious illness differ in different cultural groups? What are the effects of cultural and ethnic matching and mismatching? How do the narratives of cancer sufferers differ across different cultural groups?

Third, it has been pointed out how the psychological response to cancer varies across cultural contexts. This raises significant questions. What factors in a given culture protect against psychological disturbance in cancer? What cultural factors worsen psychological disturbance? How can coping styles be improved in different cultural groups? A related and very under-developed area is psychotherapy with ethnic minority cancer patients. Is one model of therapy useful in all cultural groups? How can different types of therapy (for instance psychodynamic or cognitive) be made more culturally appropriate and involve cultural factors? We have seen that spirituality and religion may be potent ways of coping with this disease. What aspects of a person's religious/spiritual system facilitate coping? How can religious values and ideas be incorporated into therapy? Is religion ultimately just another way of improving social support? How can religious professionals, such as chaplains, be incorporated into cancer care? Perhaps one of the most intriguing questions is whether being religious enhances mental (or possibly) physical health in those with cancer.

Fourth, the evidence that ethnic minorities receive poorer treatment for their cancer warrants further exploration. To relationships between differential treatments, access and availability of services, and the attitudes of patients and practitioners requires clarification. There is little information about how rates of uptake of treatment are tied to notions of autonomy and body image. For instance, what cultural factors relate to women choosing mastectomy as opposed to a lumpectomy where the prognoses have generally been found to be similar? There is some evidence that cancer patients resort to CAM and in some instances to traditional (often culturally congruent) healing when ill. There is a need for further understanding of why they resort to these treatments, what they gain from them and how they can be incorporated into oncology care.

Fifth, the process of dying and the response to death vary significantly across cultural groups. There is an urgent need to explore inequalities in rates of provision of palliative care. Why are uptakes of palliative care different in different groups? What role does the family play in terminal illness and how does this vary cross-culturally? Traditional and religious values play a large part in care of the dying. How can these religious and spiritual values be incorporated into terminal and hospice care? Who should provide this type of care for patients? How can ethnic minority groups be enabled to perform rituals related to death and dying in our largely secular society? Do cultural factors protect against the effects of bereavement? If so, how? Do types of grief differ among different cultural groups?

Last, a vital question relates to how cultural aspects and sensitivity could be taught to health professionals. Who are the most appropriate people to do this? What aspects should be included in a cultural competency programme? How can cultural competence be assessed and evaluated? And by whom?

The field of anthropological oncology is a slowly growing discipline. I would strongly argue that the answers to some of these research questions would greatly improve the quality of life for ethnic minority cancer sufferers and their carers and significantly reduce the severe burden that this disease presents.

References

Adams, J., White, M. and Foreman, D. (2004) Are there socio-economic gradients in stage and grade of breast cancer at diagnosis? Cross section analysis of UK cancer registry data, *British Medical Journal*, 329: 142–3.

Addington-Hall, J. (1993) *Regional Study of Care for the Dying. Feedback for District Health Authorities. Cancer Deaths Only*. London: Department of Epidemiology and Public Health, University College London.

Ahlner-Elmquist, M., Jordhoy, M., Jannert, M. *et al.* (2004) Place of death: hospital-based advanced home care versus conventional care. A prospective study in palliative cancer care, *Palliative Medicine*, 18(7): 585–93.

Ahmad, W.I.U. (1993) Making Black people sick: race, ideology and health research, in W. Ahmad (ed.) *Race & Health in Contemporary Britain*. Buckingham: Open University Press.

Ahmad, W.I.U. (1996) The trouble with culture, in D. Kelleher and S. Hillier (eds) *Researching Cultural Inequalities in Health*. London: Routledge.

Airey, C., Beecher, H., Erens, B. and Fuller, E. (2002) *National Survey of NHS Patients. Cancer: Health Overview 1999/2000*. London: Department of Health.

Aldridge, D. (1989) Europe looks at complementary therapies, *British Medical Journal*, 299: 1211–12.

Alexander, Z. (1999) *The Department of Health: Study of Black, Asian and Ethnic Minority Issues*. London: Department of Health.

American Cancer Society (1981) Black Americans' attitudes towards cancer and cancer tests: highlights of a study, *CA Cancer Journal Clinics*, 314: 212–18.

American Cancer Society (1986) *Special Report on Cancer in the Economically Disadvantaged*. Atlanta: GA American Cancer Society.

American Cancer Society (1989) *Cancer in the Poor. A Report to the Nation*. Atlanta GA: American Cancer Society.

American Cancer Society (2000) *Facts and Figures: Cancer in Minorities*. Atlanta: American Cancer Society.

American Institute for Research (2002) *Teaching Cultural Competence in Health Care: A Review of Current Concepts, Plans and Priorities*. Report prepared for the Office of Minority Health. Washington, DC: American Institute for Research.

American Society of Clinical Oncology and Cancer Research Prevention Foundation (2004) http://www.preventcancer.org/healthyliving/PreventionNews/cancerprev study.cfm

Andersen, B.L. and Cacioppo, J.T. (1995) Delay in seeking a cancer diagnosis: delay stages and psychophysiological comparison processes, *British Journal of Social Psychology*, 34: 33–52.

Arberry, A. (1994) *Discourses of Rumi*. London: Routledge.

Aries, P. (1981) *The Hour of Our Death*. New York: Oxford University Press.

Astin, J.A. (1998) Why patients use alternative medicine: results of a national study, *Journal of the American Medical Association*, 279: 1548–53.

Atkin, K. and Rollings, J. (1996) Looking after their own? Family caregiving among Asian and Afro-Caribbean communities, in W. Ahmad and K. Atkin (eds) *Race and Community Care*. Buckingham: Open University Press.

Bach, P.B., Kramer, L.D. and Warren, J.L. (1999) Racial differences in the treatment of early stage lung cancer, *New England Journal of Medicine*, 341: 1198–205.

Bach, P.B., Schrag, D., Brawley, O.W., Galaznik, A., Yakren, S. and Begg, C.B. (2002) Survival of blacks and whites after a cancer diagnosis, *Journal of the American Medical Association*, 287: 2106–13.

Bailey, E., Erwin, D. and Belam, P. (2000) Using cultural beliefs and patterns to improve mammography utilization amongst African-American women. The Witness Project, *Journal of National Medical Association*, 92: 3136–42.

Bain, R.P., Greenberg, R.S. and Whitaker, J.P. (1986) Racial differences in survival of women with breast cancer, *Journal of Chronic Diseases*, 39: 631–42.

Baker, E.H., Dong, Y.B., Sagnella, G.A. *et al.* (1998) Association of Hypertension with T594 M mutation in beta sub-unit of apical channels in black people resident in London, *Lancet*, 351: 1388–92.

Bal, P. and Bal, G. (1995) *Health Care Needs for Multi-Racial Society: A Practical Guide For Health Professionals*. London: Hawkar Publications.

Bal, S. (1987) Psychological symptomatology and health beliefs of Asian patients, in H. Dent (ed.) *Clinical Psychology: Research and Developments*. London: Croom Helm.

Balarajan, R. and Bulusu, L. (1990) Mortality among immigrants in England and Wales 1979–83, in M. Britton (ed.) *Mortality and Geography: A Review in the Mid 1980's*. London: OPCS.

Ballard-Barbash, R., Forman, M. and Kipnis, V. (1999) Dietary fat, serum oestrogen levels and breast cancer risk: a multifaceted story, *Journal of National Cancer Institute*, 91(6): 492–4.

Balshem, M. (1993) *Cancer in the Community: Class and Medical Authority*. Washington, DC: Smithsonian Series in Ethnographic Inquiry.

Bandura, A. (1977) Self-efficacy: toward a unifying theory of behavioural change, *Psychological Review*, 84: 191–213.

Barg, S. and Gullate, M. (2001) Cancer support groups – Meeting needs of African Americans with cancer, *Seminars in College Nursing*, 17(3): 171–8.

Barraclough, J. (1999) *Cancer and Emotion*. Chichester: John Wiley.

Barraclough, J. (2001) *Integrated Cancer Care: Holistic, Complementary, and Creative Approaches*. Oxford: Oxford University Press.

Baxter, C. (1989) Cancer support and ethnic minority and migrant worker communities. Unpublished paper.

Beauchamp, T. and Childress, J. (2001) *Principles of Biomedical Ethics*, 5th edn. Oxford: Oxford University Press.

Beck, U. and Beck-Gernsheim, E. (2002) *Individualisation: Institutionalised Individualism and its Social and Political Consequences*. London: Sage.

Bergum, V. (1989) Being a phenomenological researcher, in J. Morse (ed.) *Qualitative Nursing Research: A Contemporary Dialogue*. London: Sage Publications.

Bezwoda, W., Colvin, H. and Lehoka, J. (1997) Transcultural and language problems in communicating with cancer patients in southern Africa, *Annals New York Academy of Science*, 809: 119–32.

Bhakta, P., Donnelly, P. and Mayberry, J. (1995) Management of breast disease in Asian women, *Professional Nursing*, 11: 187–9.

Bhal, V. (1996) Cancer in ethnic minorities: Department of Health perspective, *British Journal of Cancer Supplement*, 29: S2–10.

Bhopal, R. (1986) The interrelationship of folk, traditional and western medicine within an Asian community in Britain, *Social Science and Medicine*, 22: 99–105.

Bhopal, R. (1997) Research into ethnicity and health races, unsound or important science, *British Medical Journal*, 314: 1751–6.

Bhopal, R. (2001) Ethnicity and race as epidemiological variables: sensuality of purpose and context, in H. Macbeth and P. Shetty (eds) *Health and Ethnicity*. London: Taylor & Francis.

Bhopal, R. and Rankin, J. (1996) Cancer in minority ethnic populations, *British Journal of Cancer* Supplement, 74: S522–532.

Bigby, J. and Perez-Sable, E. (2004) The challenges of understanding and eliminating racial and ethnic disparities in health, *Journal of General Internal Medicine*, 19: 201–3.

Blackhall, L.J., Frank, G., Murphy, S.T. *et al.* (1999) Ethnicity and attitudes towards life sustaining technology, *Social Science and Medicine*, 48: 1779–89.

Blackhall, L., Murphy, S., Frank, G. *et al.* (1995) Ethnicity and attitudes toward patient autonomy, *Journal of American Medical Association*, 274(10): 820–5.

Bodell, J. and Weng, M.A. (2000) The Jewish patient and terminal dehydration: a hospice ethical dilemma, *American Journal of Hospice and Palliative Care*, 17(3): 185–8. Review.

Bonham, V. (2001) Race, ethnicity and pain treatment: striving to understand the causes and solutions to the disparities in pain treatment, *Journal of Law and Medical Ethics*, 291: 52–68.

Boon, H., Bell-Brown, J., Gavin, A. and Westlake, K. (2003) Men with prostate cancer: making decisions about complementary alternative medicine, *Medical Decision Making*, 23(6): 471–9.

Boon, H., Brown, J.B., Gavin, A. *et al.* (1999) Breast cancer survivors' perceptions of complementary/alternative medicine (CAM): making the decision to use or not to use, *Qualitative Health Research*, 9: 639–53.

Bottorff, J.L., Johnson, J.L., Bhagat, R. *et al.* (1998) Beliefs related to breast health practices: the perceptions of South Asian women living in Canada, *Social Science and Medicine*, 47: 2075–85.

Bowling, J. (1995) Guinea across the water: the African American approach to death and dying, in J. Perry and A. Ryan (eds) *A Cross Cultural Look at Death, Dying and Religion*. Chicago, Ill: Nelson Hall.

Box, B. (1984) Cancer and misconceptions, *Journal of the Royal Society of Health*, 104: 161–70.

Brady, M.J., Peterman, A.H., Fitchett, G. *et al.* (1999) A case for including spirituality in quality of life measurement in oncology, *Psychooncology*, 8(5): 417–28.

Broman, C.L. (1996) Coping with personal problems, in H.W. Neighbors and J.S. Jackson (eds) *Mental Health in Black America*. Thousand Oaks, CA: Sage.

Bronfen, E. (1992) *Over Her Dead body: Death, Femininity and the Aesthetic*. Manchester: Manchester University Press.

Brown, J., Byers, T., Doyle, C. *et al.* (2003) Nutrition and physical activity during and after cancer treatment: an American Cancer Society guide for informed choices, *CA: A Cancer Journal for clinicians*, 53: 268–91.

Bruera, E., Neumann, C., Mazzocato, C., Stiefel, F. and Sala, R. (2000) Attitudes and beliefs of palliative care physicians regarding communication with terminally ill cancer patients, *Palliative Medicine*, 14: 287–98.

Bulatao, R. and Stephens, P. (1991) Estimates and projections of mortality by cause: a global overview 1970–2015, in D. Jamison and H. Mosley (eds) *The World Bank Health Sector Priorities Review*. Washington DC: World Bank.

Bulka, R. (1998) *Judaism on Illness and Suffering*. New York: Jason Aronson.

Bullinger, M., Anderson, R., Cella, D. and Aaronson, N. (1993) Developing and evaluating cross-cultural instruments from minimum requirements to optimal models, *Quality of Life Research*, 2(6): 451–9.

Burgess, C., Ramirez, A. and Love, S. (1998) Who and what influences delayed presentation in breast cancer, *British Journal of Cancer*, 77: 1343–8.

Burhanssitpanov, L. (2000) Urban Native American health issues, *Cancer*, 88(5Suppl): 1207–13.

Burke, C. and Sikora, K. (1993) Complementary and conventional cancer care: the integration of two cultures, *Clinical Oncology*, 5: 220–7.

Bush, J., White, M., Kai, J. and Bhopal, R. (2003) Understanding influences on smoking in Bangladeshi and Pakistani adults: community based, qualitative study, *British Medical Journal*, 326(7396): 962.

Butow, P., Kazemi, J., Beeney, L. *et al.* (1996) When the diagnosis is cancer: communication experiences and preferences, *Cancer*, 77(12): 2630–7.

Calman, K. and Hine, D. (1995) *A Policy Framework for Commissioning Cancer Services – Report by the Expert Advisory Group on Cancer to the Chief Medical Officers of England and Wales*. (Calman/Hine Report). London: Department of Health.

Cancer Research Campaign (1996) The proceedings of the Cancer Research Campaign/Department of Health Symposium on Ethnic Minorities and Cancer, *British Journal of Cancer*, (Suppl.) Sep 29, s1–82.

Cancer Research UK (2004) *Information Resource Centre*.

Carlick, A. and Biley, F. (2004) Thoughts on the therapeutic use of narrative in the promotion of coping in cancer care, *European Journal of Cancer Care*, 13(4): 308.

Carpenter, J.S., Brockopp, D.Y. and Andrykowski, M.A. (1999) Self-transformation as a factor in the self-esteem and well-being of breast cancer survivors, *Journal of Advanced Nursing*, 29(6): 1402–11.

Carver, C.S., Pozo, C., Harris, S.D. *et al.* (1993) How coping mediates the effect of optimism on distress: a study of women with early stage breast cancer, in R. Suinn and G. Vandenbos (eds) *Cancer Patients and Their Families: Readings on Disease Course, Coping, and Psychological Interventions.* Washington, DC: APA Books.

Cassell, E. (1982) The nature of suffering and the goals of medicine. *New England Journal of Medicine,* 306: 639–45.

Cassileth, B., Lusk, E. and Guerry, D. (1991) Survival and quality of life among patients receiving unproven as compared with unconventional cancer therapy. *New England Journal of Medicine,* 324: 1180–5.

Cassileth, B., Lusk, E. and Strouse, T. (1984) Contemporary unorthodox treatment in cancer medicine: a study of patients' treatment and practitioners, *Annals of Internal Medicine,* 101: 105–12.

Centeno-Cortes, C. and Nun-Olarte, J. (1994) Questioning diagnosis disclosure in terminal cancer patients: a prospective study evaluating patients' responses. *Palliative Medicine,* 8: 39–44.

Chambers, T. (2000) Cross cultural issues in caring for patients with cancer, *Cancer Treatment Research,* 102: 23–37.

Charlton, R. and Dovey, S. (1995) Attitudes to death and dying in the UK, New Zealand and Japan, *Journal of Palliative Care,* 11: 42–7.

Chattoo, S., Ahmad, W., Haworth, M. *et al.* (2002) *South Asian and White Patients with Advanced Cancer: Patients' and Families' Experiences of the Illness and Perceived Needs for Care* (final Report to CRC UK and the Department of Health). Leeds: Centre for Research in Primary care, University of Leeds.

Chaturvedi, S.K. (1994) Exploration of concerns and role of psychosocial intervention in palliative care: a study from India, *Annals Academic Medicine Singapore,* 23: 256–60.

Chavez, L.R., Hubbell, F.A., McMullin, J.M. *et al.* (1995) Structure and meaning of models of breast and cervical cancer risk factors: a comparison of perceptions among Latinas, Anglo women and physicians, *Medical Anthropology Quarterly,* 9: 40–74.

Chavez, L., Hubbell, F. and Mishra, S. (1999) Ethnography and breast cancer control among Latinas and Anglo women in Southern California, in R. Hahn (ed.) *Anthropology in Public Health: Bridging Differences in Culture and Society.* New York: Oxford University Press.

Chavez, L.R., Hubbell, F.A., Mishra, S.I. and Valdez, R.B. (1997) The influence of fatalism on self-reported use of papanicolau smears, *American Journal of Preventative Medicine,* 13: 418–24.

Cherny, N. (1998) Cancer pain: principles of assessment and syndromes, in A. Berger, R. Portenoy and D. Weissman (eds) *Supportive Care.* Philadelphia: Lippincott-Raven.

Chiu, L.F. (2003) Health promotion and screening, in J. Kai (ed.) *Ethnicity, Health and Primary Care.* Oxford: Oxford University Press.

Chochinov, H. and Breitbart, W. (2000) *Handbook of Psychiatry in Palliative Medicine.* Oxford: Oxford University Press.

Choudhry, U., Srivastava, R. and Fitch, M. (1998) Breast cancer detection practices of south Asian women: knowledge, attitudes, and beliefs, *Oncology Nursing Forum,* 25(10): 1693–1701.

Christakis, M. (2000) *Death Foretold: Prophecy and Prognosis in Medical Care*. Chicago, Ill: University of Chicago Press.

Christman, N. and Johnson, T. (1990) Clinically applied anthropology, in T. Johnson and C. Sargent (eds) *Medical Anthropology: A Handbook of Theory and Method*. New York: Greenwood Press.

Chvetzoff, G. and Tannock, I. (2003) Placebo effects on oncology, *Journal of the National Cancer Institute*, 95(1): 19–29.

CIOMS (Council for International Organisations of Medical Sciences) and (WHO) World Health Organisation (1993) *International Ethical Guidelines for Biomedical Research Involving Human Subjects*. Proposed Guidelines, 1983. Revised and adopted, 2002. Geneva: CIOMS/WHO.

Cleeland, C.S., Gonin, R., Baez, L., Loehrer, P. and Pandya, K. (1997) Pain and treatment of pain in minority patients with cancer. The Eastern Cooperative Oncology Group Minority Outpatient Pain Study, *Annals of Internal Medicine*, 127(9): 813–16.

Cleeland, C.S., Gonin, R., Hatfield, A.K. *et al.* (1994) Pain and its treatment in outpatients with metastatic cancer, *New England Journal of Medicine*, 330: 592–6.

Cline, S. (1995) *Lifting the Taboo: Women, Death and Dying*. London: Little Brown and Co.

Coates, R.J., Bransfield, D.D., Wellesley, M. *et al.* (1992) Differences between black and white women with breast cancer in time from symptom recognition to medical consultation. Black/White Cancer Survival Study Group, *Journal of the National Cancer Institute*, 84: 938–50.

Cobb, M. (2001) *The Dying Soul: Spiritual Care At The End Of Life*. Buckingham: Open University Press.

Colditz, G. and Gortmaker, S. (1995) Cancer prevention strategies for the future: risk intervention and preventive intervention, *Millbank Q*, 73(4): 621–51.

Coleman-Miller, B. (2000) A physician's perspective on minority health, *Healthcare Financing and Review*, 214: 45–56.

Conrad, M., Brown, P. and Conrad, M. (1996) Fatalism and breast cancer in Black women, *Annals of Internal Medicine*, 125(11): 141–2.

Cooley, M.E. and Jennings-Dozier, K. (1998) Cultural assessment of Black American men treated for prostate cancer: clinical case studies, *Oncology Nursing Forum*, 25: 1729–36.

Cooper, H., Lester, H. and Wilson, S. (2003) Representation of South Asian people in randomised trials, *British Medical Journal*, 327: 394–5.

Cooper-Patrick, L., Gallo, J.J., Gonzales, J.J. *et al.* (1999) Race, gender, and partnership in the patient–physician relationship, *Journal of the American Medical Association*, 282: 583–9.

Corbie-Smith, G., Miller, W. and Ransohoff, M. (2004) Interpretations of 'appropriate' minority inclusion clinical research, *American Journal of Medicine*, 116(4): 249–52.

Coss, A., McGrath, P. and Thegiano, V. (1998) Alternative Care. Patient choices for adjunct therapies within the cancer centre, *Cancer Practice*, 6: 176–81.

Costantini, M., Camoirano, E., Madeddu, L. *et al.* (1993) Palliative home care and place of death among cancer patients: a population based survey, *Palliative Medicine*, 7: 323–31.

Coulter, I. and Willis, E. (2004) The rise and rise of complementary alternative medicine: a sociological perspective, *The Medical Journal of Australia*, 180(11): 587–9.

Crawford, R. (1980) Healthism and the medicalisation of everyday life, *International Journal of Health Services*, 19: 365–88.

Crawley, L. and La Vera, M. (2002) Palliative care in African American communities, *Journal of Palliative Medicine*, 5(5): 775–9.

Crawley, L., Payne, R., Bolden, J. *et al.* (2000) Palliative and end-of-life care in the African American community, *JAMA*, 284: 2518–21.

Crocetti, E., Crotti, N., Feltrin, A. *et al.* (1998) The use of complementary therapies for breast cancer patients attending conventional treatment, *European Journal of Cancer*, 34: 324–8.

Crook, S., Pakulski, S. and Waters, M. (1998) *Post Modernisation: Changes in Advanced Society*. London: Sage.

Cross, T., Bazron, B., Dennis, K.W. and Isaacs, M.R. (1989) *Towards a Culturally Competent System of Care*, Volume I. Washington, DC: Georgetown University Child Development Center: CASSP Technical Assistance Center.

Culver, J.L., Arena, P.L., Antoni, M.H. and Carver, C.S. (2002) Coping and distress among women under treatment for early stage breast cancer: comparing African Americans, Hispanics and non-Hispanic whites, *Psych-Oncology*, 11: 495–504.

Davis, J. and Smith, T. (1990) *General Social Survey 1972–1990*. Chicago National Opinion Research Centre.

Davison, C., Frankel, S. and Davey Smith, G. (1992) The limits of lifestyle: re-assessing 'fatalism' in the popular culture of illness prevention, *Social Science and Medicine*, 34: 675–85.

Dein, S. (2003) Mind-body therapies and the psycho-oncology debate. *European Journal of Palliative Care*, 103: 30–2.

Dein, S. (2004a) Explanatory models and attitudes towards cancer in different cultures, *Lancet Oncology*, 5: 119–24.

Dein, S. (2004b) Working with patients with religious beliefs, *Advances in Psychiatric Treatment*, 10: 287–95.

Dein, S. (2004c) From chaos to cosmogeny: a comparison of understandings of the narrative process among Western academics and Hasidic Jews, *Anthropology and Medicine*, 11(2): 135–47.

Dein, S. (2005) Attitudes towards cancer among elderly Bangladeshis in London, *European Journal of Cancer Care*, 14(2): 149–50.

Dein, S. (in press) Race, culture and ethnicity in ethnic minority research: a critical discussion, *Journal of Cultural Diversity*.

Dein, S. and Bhui, K. (2005) Informed consent for medical research among non-westernised ethnic minority patients: a discussion paper, *Journal of the Royal Society of Medicine*, 98: 354–6.

Dein, S. and Thomas, K. (2002) To tell or not to tell: cultural and religious factors related to the disclosure of a fatal prognosis, *European Journal of Palliative Care*, 9(5): 209–12.

Department of Health (2004) *National Survey of NHS Patients: Cancer: Analysis of Themes*. London: DoH.

DHSS (2001) www.healthgap.omhrc.gov/hgfs.htm

Dibble, S.L., Vanoni, J.M. and Miaskowski, C. (1997) Women's attitudes toward breast cancer screening procedures: differences by ethnicity, *Women's Health Issues*, 7: 47–54.

Diversity Resources Inc. (2001) *Culture Sensitive Health Care: American Indian.* Blacksburg: VA Virginia Tech, Office of Multicultural Affairs. Diversity and Work/ Life Resource Center.

Dodd, M., Chan, N., Lindsey, A. and Piper, B. (1985) Attitudes of patients living in Taiwan about cancer and its treatment, *Cancer Nursing*, 8: 214–20.

Dogra, N. (2001) The development and evaluation of a program to teach cultural diversity to medical undergraduate students, *Medical Education*, 35(3): 232–41.

Dogra, N., Connin, S., Gill, P., Spencer, J. and Turner, M. (2005) Teaching of cultural diversity in medical schools in the United Kingdom and the Republic of Ireland: cross sectional questionnaire survey, *British Medical Journal*, 330: 403–4.

Donovan, J. (1986) *We Don't Buy Sickness. It Just Comes.* London: Gower.

Downer, S.M., Cody, M.M., McCluskey, P. *et al.* (1994) Pursuit and practice of complementary therapies by cancer patients receiving conventional treatment, *British Medical Journal*, 309: 86–9.

Doyley, Y. (1991) A survey of the cervical screening service in a London district, including reasons for non attendance, ethnic responses and views on the quality of the service, *Social Science and Medicine*, 32: 953–7.

Duminda, R., Weed, D. and Shankar, S. (1999) Cancer knowledge and misconceptions amongst immigrant Salvadorian men in the Washington DC area, *Journal of Immigrant Health*, 1: 207–13.

Duncan, V., Parrott, R. and Silk, K. (2001) African American women's perceptions of the role of genetics in breast cancer risk, *American Journal of Health Studies*, 172: 50–8.

Dunlop, R., Daviews, R. and Hockley, J. (1989) Preferred vs actual place of death: a hospital palliative care support team study, *Palliative Medicine*, 3: 197–201.

Durfy, S., Bowen, D., McTieman, A. and Sporleder, J. (1999) Attitudes and interest in genetic testing for breast and ovarian cancer susceptibility in diverse groups of women in Western Washington, *Cancer Epidemiology, Biomarkers and Prevention*, 8: 369–75.

Eastwood, H. (2000) Why are Australian GPs using alternative medicine? Post modernisation, consumerism and the shift towards holistic health, *Journal of Sociology*, 36: 133–56.

Ebrahim, S. (1996) Ethnic elders, *British Medical Journal*, 313: 610–13.

Edwards, B., Howe, H., Ries, L. *et al.* (2002) Annual report to the nation on the status of cancer, 1973–1999, featuring implications of age and aging on US cancer burden, *Cancer*, 94(10): 2766–92.

Eisenberg, D.M., Kessler, R.C., Foster, C. *et al.* (1993) Unconventional medicine in the United States, *New England Journal of Medicine*, 328: 246–52.

Eisenbruch, M. (1984) Cross-cultural aspects of bereavement. II: ethnic and cultural variations in the development of bereavement practices, *Cultural, Medicine and Psychiatry*, 84: 315–47.

El Sarag, H. (2002) Hepatocellular carcinoma: an epidemiologic view, *Journal of Clinical Gastroenterology*, 35 (supp 2): 72–8.

Ell, K. and Nishimoto, R. (1989) Coping resources in adaptation to cancer-analysis of socio-economic and racial differences, *Social Services Review*, 63: 443–6.

Ernst, E. (1995) Complementary medicine: what physicians think of it: a meta analysis, *Archives of Internal Medicine*, 155(22): 2405–8.

Ernst, E. (2000) The role of complementary and alternative medicine, *British Medical Journal*, 321: 1133–5.

Ernst, E. and Cassileth, B.R. (1998) The prevalence of complementary/alternative medicine in cancer: a systematic review, *Cancer*, 83: 777–82.

Ernst, E., Resch, K., Hill, R. *et al.* (1995) Complementary medicine – a definition. *British Journal of General Practice* 45: 506.

Ernst, E. and White, A. (2000) The BBC survey of complementary medicine in the UK, *Complementary Therapies in Medicine*, 8: 32–6.

Erwin, D.O. (1987) The militarisation of cancer treatment in American society, in H.A. Baer (ed.) *Encounters with Biomedicine: Case Studies in Medical Anthropology*. New York: Gordon and Breach.

Eskandari, F. and Sternberg, E. (2002) Neural-immune interactions in health and disease, *New York Academy of Sciences*, 966: 20–7.

Eve, A., Smith, A. and Tebbit, P. (1997) Hospice and palliative care in the UK 1994–95, including a summary of trends 1990–95, *Palliative Medicine*, 11: 31–43.

Faass, N. (2001) *Integrating Complementary Medicine into Health Systems*. Gaithersburg: Aspen Publications.

Facione, N.C., Dodd, M.J., Holzemer, W. and Meleis, A.I. (1997) Help seeking for self-discovered breast symptoms. Implications for early detection, *Cancer Practice*, 5: 220–7.

Facione, N.C., Giancarlo, C. and Chan, L. (2000) Perceived risk and help-seeking behaviour for breast cancer. A Chinese-American perspective, *Cancer Nursing*, 23: 258–67.

Fallowfield, L. (1997) Truth sometimes hurts but deceit hurts more, *Annals of the New York Academy of Science*, 809: 525–36.

Fallowfield, L., Ford, S. and Lewis, S. (1995) No news is not good news: information preferences of patients with cancer, *Psycho-oncology*, 4: 197–202.

Fallowfield, L., Rodway, A. and Baum, M. (1990) What are the psychological factors influencing attendance, non attendance and reattendance at a breast screening centre? *Journal of Royal Society of Medicine*, 83: 547–51.

Fassil, J. (1996) *Primary Health Care for Black and Minority Ethnic People: A Consumer Perspective*. Leeds: NHS Ethnic Health Unit.

Feeland, M. and Parkman, S. (1995) How to do it: work with an interpreter, *British Medical Journal*, 311: 555–7.

Ferlay, J., Bray, F., Pisani, P. and Parkin, D.M. (2004) GLOBOCAN 2002: *Cancer Incidence, Mortality and Prevalence Worldwide*. Lyon: IARC Press.

Field, D. (1998) Special not different: general practitioners' accounts of their care of dying people. *Social Science and Medicine*, 46: 1111–20.

Field, D. and Copp, G. (1999) Communication and awareness about dying in the 1990s, *Palliative Medicine*, 13: 459–568.

Field, D., Hockey, J. and Small, N. (1997) *Death, Gender and Ethnicity*. London: Routledge.

Firth, S. (1993a) Cultural issues in terminal care, in D. Clark (ed.) *The Future of Palliative Care: Issues of Policy and Practice*. Buckingham: Open University Press.

Firth, S. (1993b) Approaches to death in Hindu and Sikh communities in Britain, in D. Dickenson and M. Johnson (eds) *Death, Dying and Bereavement*. London: Sage.

Firth, S. (1996) 'The good death': attitudes of British Hindus, in G. Howarth and P. Jupp (eds) *Contemporary Issues in the Sociology of Death, Dying and Disposal*. Basingstoke: Macmillan.

Firth, S. (1997) *Dying, Death and Bereavement in a British Hindu Community*. Leuven: Peeters.

Firth, S. (2001) *Wider Horizons*. London: National Council for Hospice and Specialist Palliative Care Services.

Fisher, P. and Ward, A. (1994) Complementary medicine in Europe, *British Medical Journal*, 309: 107–11.

Flood, A., Velie, E., Chatergee, N. *et al.* (2002) Fruit and vegetable intakes and the risk of colorectal cancer in the Breast Cancer Detection Demonstration Project follow-up cohort, *American Journal of Clinical Nutrition*, 75(5): 936–43.

Flores, G., Gee, D. and Kastner, B. (2000) The teaching of cultural issues in US and Canadian medical schools, *Academic Medicine*, 5(75): 541–55.

Fontaine, K. and Smith, S. (1995) Optimistic bias in cancer risk perception: a cross-national study, *Psychological Reports*, 77: 143–6.

Foster, G. and Anderson, B. (1978) *Medical Anthropology*. New York: Wiley.

Foster, R.S. and Costanza, M.C. (1984) Breast self-examination practices and breast cancer survival, *Cancer*, 53: 999–1005.

Fountain, A. (1999) Ethnic minorities in Derby, *Palliative Medicine*, 13: 161–2.

Frank, A. (1997) *The Wounded Story Teller: Body Illness and Ethics*. Chicago: Chicago University Press.

Freeman, H. (1989) Cancer in the socioeconomically disadvantaged, *Cancer*, 39: 266–88.

Freeman, H. (2004) Poverty, culture and social injustice: cancer disparities. *Cancer Journal Clinics*, 54: 72–7.

Frisby, C. (2002) Messages of hope: health communication strategies that address barriers preventing black women from screening for breast cancer, *Journal of Black Studies*, 325: 489–505.

Fuller, J. (2003) Effective cross-cultural communication, in J. Kai (ed.) *Ethnicity, Health and Primary Care: A Practical Guide*. Oxford: Oxford University Press.

Garfinkel, L. and Mushinski, M. (1999) US cancer incidence mortality and survival 1973–1996, *Statistical Bulletin of Metropolitan Insurance Companies*, 80: 23–32.

Gattellari, M., Voigt, K., Butow, P. and Tattersall, M. (2002) When the treatment goal is not cure: are cancer patients equipped to make informed decisions? *Journal of Clinical Oncology*, 20(2): 503–13.

Geiger, H. (2001) Racial stereotyping and medicine: the need for cultural competence, *Canadian Medical Association Journal*, 164(12): 1699–70.

Gemson, D.H., Elinson, J. and Messeri, P. (1988) Differences in physician preventive practice pattern for white and minority patients, *Journal of Community Health*, 13: 53–64.

Georgaki, S., Kalaidopoulou, O., Liarmakopoulos, I. and Mystakidou, K. (2002) Nurses' attitudes toward truthful communication with patients with cancer. A Greek study, *Cancer Nursing*, 256: 436–41.

Germino, B.B., Mishel, M.H., Belyea, M. *et al.* (1998) Uncertainty in prostate cancer. Ethnic and family patterns, *Cancer Practice*, 62: 107–13.

Ghafoor, A., Jemal, A. and Cokkinides, V. (2002) Cancer statistics for African Americans, *CA A Cancer Journal for Clinicians*, 52: 326–41.

Gibson, C., Pessin, H., McLain, C. *et al.* (2004) The unmet need : addressing spirituality and meaning through culturally sensitive communication and intervention, in R. Moore and D. Spiegel *Cancer, Culture and Communication*. New York: Kluwer Academic/Plenum Publishers.

Gifford, S. (1994) The change of life, the sorrow of life: menopause, bad blood and cancer among Italian-Australian working class women, *Culture, Medicine and Psychiatry*, 18: 299–314.

Gill, P., Kai, J., Bhopal, R. and Wilde, S. (2003) Health care needs assessment of black and ethnic minority groups, in J. Raftery, J. Mant and A. Stevens (eds) *The Epidemiologically Based Health Needs Assessment Reviews*. Third Series. Abingdon: Radcliffe.

Ginsberg, M., Quirt, C., Ginsberg, A. and MacKillop, W. (1995) Psychiatric illness and psychosocial concerns of patients with newly diagnosed lung cancer, *Canadian Medical Association Journal*, 152: 701–8.

Giuliano, A., Papenfuss, M., Schneider, A., Nour, M. and Hatch, K. (1999) Risk factors for high-risk type human papilloma virus among Mexican-American women, *Cancer Epidemiology Biomarkers Prevention*, 8(7): 615–20.

Glanz, K. (2003) *Cancer in Women of Colour Monograph*. Bethesda MD: US Department of Health and Human Services. National Cancer Institute.

Glanz, K., Grove, J., Lerman, C., Gotay, C. and Le Marchand, L. (1999) Correlates of intentions to obtain genetic counselling and colorectal cancer gene testing among at risk relatives from three ethnic groups, *Cancer Epidemiology, Biomarkers & Prevention*, 8: 329–36.

Goh, C.R., Lee, K.S., Tan, T.C. *et al.* (1996) Measuring quality of life in different cultures: translation of the functional living index for cancer SOIC in China, Malaya and Singapore, *Annals Academic Medicine Singapore*, 25: 323–34.

Goldstein, D., Thewes, B. and Butow, P. (2002) Communicating in a multi-cultural society 2: Greek community attitudes towards cancer in Australia, *Internal Medicine Journal*, 32: 289–96.

Good, B. (1994) *Medicine, Rationality and Experience: An Anthropological Perspective*. Cambridge: Cambridge University Press.

Good, M.J.D., Good, B.J., Schaffer, C. and Lind, S.E. (1990) American oncology and discourse of hope, *Culture, Medicine and Psychiatry*, 14: 59–79.

Gordon, A. (1996) Hospice and minorities: a national study of organisational access and practice, *The Hospice Journal*, 11(1): 49–70.

Gordon, D.R. and Paci, E. (1997) Disclosure practices and cultural narratives: understanding concealment and silence around cancer in Tuscany, Italy, *Social Science and Medicine*, 44: 1433–52.

Gregg, J. and Curry, R. (1994) Explanatory models for cancer amongst African American Women at two Atlanta neighbouring health centres: the implications of cancer screening programme, *Social Science and Medicine*, 39: 519–26.

Gregorio, D., Cummmings, R.M. and Michalek, K.A. (1983) Delay, stage of disease and survival among white and black women with breast cancer, *American Journal of Public Health*, 73: 590–3.

Greiner, K., Perera, S. and Ahluwalia, J. (2003) Hospice usage by minorities in the last year of life: results from the National Mortality Followback Survey, *Journal of American Geriatric Society*, 51: 970–8.

Grossfield, G.D., Latini, D.M., Downs, T. *et al.* (2002) Is ethnicity an independent predictor of prostate cancer recurrence after radical prostatectomy? *Journal of Urology*, 168(6): 2510–15.

Grothey, A., Deep, J., Hasenburg, A. and Viogtmann, R. (1998) Anwendung Alternativ Medizinischer Methoden Durch Klogische Patienten. *DTSH MED WSCHR*, 123: 923–9.

Grunfeld, E., Ramirez, A., Hunter, M. and Richards, M. (2002) Women's knowledge and beliefs regarding breast cancer, *British Journal of Cancer*, 869: 1373–8.

Gunaratnam, Y. (1997) Culture is not enough, in D. Field, J. Hockey, N. Small (eds) *Death, Gender and Ethnicity*. London: Routledge.

Haber, D. (1999) Minority access to hospice, *American Journal of Hospice and Palliative Care*, 16(1): 386–9.

Hahn, R. (1997) The Nocebo Phenomenon: concept, evidence and implications of public health, *Preventive Medicine*, 26(5): 607–11.

Hahn, R. (1999) *Anthropology in Public Health: Bridging Differences in Culture and Society*. New York: Oxford University Press.

Hall, S. and Rockhill, B. (2002) Race, poverty, affluence and breast cancer, *American Journal of Public Health*, 92(10): 1559; author reply: 1560.

Harding, S. and Rosato, M. (1999) Cancer incidence among first generation Scottish, Irish, West Indian and South Asian immigrants living in England and Wales, *Ethnicity and Health*, 4(1–2): 83–92.

Haroon-Iqbal, H., Field, D., Parker, H. and Iqbal, Z. (1995) The absent minority: access and use of palliative care services by black and ethnic minority groups in Leicester, in A. Richardson and J. Wilson-Barnett (eds) *Research in Cancer Nursing*. London: Scutari.

Harper, B.C. (1995) Report from the national task force and access to hospice care by minority groups, *The Hospice Journal*, 10(2): 1–9.

Harvie, M. (2003) Central obesity and breast cancer risk: a systematic review, *Obesity Reviews*, 4: 157–73.

Hawthorne, K. (1994) Accessibility and the use of healthcare services in the British Asian community, *Family Practice*, 11: 453–9.

Hay, L. (1989) *Heal Your Body: The Mental Causes for Physical Illness and the Metaphysical Way to Overcome Them*. London: Eden Grove.

Haynes, M. and Smedley, B. (1999) *The Unequal Burden of Cancer: An Assessment of NIH Research and Programs for Ethnic Minorities and the Medically Underserved*. Washington, DC: National Academy Press.

Health Development Agency (2000) *Tobacco and England's Ethnic Minorities*. London HDA.

Health Education Authority (2000) *Black and Minority Ethnic Groups in England.* London: HEA.

Helman, C. (2001) *Culture, Health and Illness.* London: Hodder Arnold.

Henderson, P.D., Gore, S.V., Davis, B.L. and Condon, E.H. (2003) African American women coping with breast cancer: a qualitative analysis, *Oncology Nursing Forum*, 30(4): 641–7.

Henley, A. (1987) *Caring in a Multi-Cultural Society.* London: Bloomsbury Health Authority.

Henschke, U.K., Leffall, L.D. Jr, Mason, C.H. *et al.* (1973) Alarming increase of the cancer mortality in the US black population (1950–1967), *Cancer*, 31: 753–68.

Hertz, R. (1960) A contribution to the study of the collective representation of death, in *Death and the Right Hand.* Glencoe: The Free Press.

Herzlich, C. and Pierret, J. (1987) *Illness and Self in Society.* Baltimore, CA: Johns Hopkins University Press.

Hill, D. and Penso, D. (1995) *Opening Doors – Improving Access to Hospice and Specialist Palliative Care Services by Members of Black and Ethnic Minority Communities.* Occasional Paper 7. London: NCHSPCS.

Hill, J., Wyatt, H., Reed, G. and Peters, J. (2003) Obesity and the environment: where do we go from here? *Science*, 299: 853–5.

Hinton, J. (1963) The physical and mental distress of the dying, *Quarterly Journal of Medicine*, 32: 1–21.

Hinton, J. (1991) *Dying.* Harmondsworth: Penguin.

Hoare, T. (1996) Breast screening and ethnic minorities, *British Journal of Cancer Supplement*, 29: S38–41.

Hockey, J.L. (1990) *Experiences of Death: An Anthropological Account.* Edinburgh: Edinburgh University Press.

Honda, K. (2003) Who gets the information about genetic testing for cancer risk? The role of race/ethnicity, immigration status, and primary care physicians, *Clinical Genetics*, 64: 131–6.

Horwitz, R. and Horwitz, S. (1993) Adherence to treatment. Health outcomes, *Archives of Internal Medicine*, 153: 1863–8.

Hsu, F. (1971) Psychosocial homeostasis. Conceptual tools for advancing psychological anthropology, *American Anthropologist*, 73: 23–44.

Huang, X., Butow, P. and Meiser, M. (1999) Attitudes and information needs of Chinese migrant cancer patients and their relatives, *Australian & New Zealand Journal of Medicine*, 29(2): 207–13.

Hughes, C., Gomez-Caminero, A., Benkendorf, J. *et al.* (1997) Ethnic differences in knowledge and attitudes about BRAC1 testing in women at increased risk, *Patient Education Counselling*, 32: 51–62.

Hunt, M. (2001) Exploring the repressive coping styles of non-Hispanic white and African American with newly diagnosed stage 2 and recurrent breast cancer. The impact of religiosity and under-reporting stressful life events, *Dissertation Abstracts International*, section B of Sciences and Engineering 62 (3) – B 1580.

Hussain-Gambles, M., Leese, B., Atkin Brown, J., Mason, S. and Tovey, P. (2004) Involving South Asian patients in clinical trials, *Health Technology Assessment*, 8(42): 73–9.

IARC (International Agency for Research on Cancer) (2002) World Health

Organisation (WHO). *IARC Handbook of Cancer Prevention, Weight Control and Physical Activity*, Vol 6. Lyon: IARC Press.

Infeld, D., Gordon, A. and Harper, B. (1995) *Hospice Care and Cultural Diversity*. New York: Haworth Press.

Institute of Medicine (1999) *The Unequal Burden of Cancer*. Washington, DC: National Academy Press.

Institute of Medicine (2003) *Unequal Treatment Confronting Racial and Ethnic Disparities in Healthcare*. Washington, DC: National Academy Press.

Iqbal, H.H., Field, D., Parker, H. and Iqbal, Z. (1995) The absent minority: access and use of palliative care services by Black and minority ethnic groups in Leicester, in A. Richardson and J. Wilson-Barnett (eds).

Jablensky, A., Sartorius, N., Gulbinet, W. and Ernberg, G. (1981) Characteristics of depressive patients connecting psychiatric services in four cultures. A report from the WHO collaborative study on the assessment of depressive disorders, *Acta Psychiatrica Scandanavia*, 63: 367–83.

Jack, C., Penny, L. and Nazar, W. (2001) Effective palliative care for minority ethnic groups – the role of a liaison worker, *International Journal of Palliative Nursing*, 7: 375–440.

Jemal, A., Thomas, A., Murray, T. *et al.* (2002) *Cancer Statistics* 2002 CA 52(1): 23–48.

Jenkins, R. and Pargament, K. (1988) Cognitive appraisals in cancer patients, *Social Science and Medicine*, 26: 625–33.

Jennings, K. (1996) Getting Black women to screen for cancer: incorporating health beliefs into practice, *Journal of The American Academy of Nurse Practitioners*, 8: 53–9.

Johnson, J., Bottorff, J. and Balneaves, L. (1999) South Asian women's views on the cause of breast cancer: images and explanations, *Patient Education Counselling*, 373: 243–54.

Johnson, S. and Spilka, B. (1991) Coping with breast cancer: the roles of clergy and faith, *Journal of Religion and Health*, 20: 21–33.

Jones, D. and Gill, P. (2003) Interpreting and translation, in J. Kai (ed.) *Ethnicity, Health, Primary care*. Oxford: Oxford University Press.

Jones, J.H. (1993) *Bad Blood: The Tuskegee Experiment*. New York: Free Press.

Jonker, G. (1996) 'The knife's edge: Muslim burial in the diaspora', *Mortality*, 1(1): 27–43.

Kaczorowski, J. (1989) Spiritual well-being and anxiety in adults diagnosed with cancer, *Hospice Journal*, 5: 105–16.

Kagawa-Singer, M., Wellisch, D.K. and Durvasula, R. (1997) Impact of breast cancer on Asian American, and Anglo American women, *Culture, Medicine and Psychiatry*, 21: 449–80.

Kai, J. (2003) *Ethnicity, Health and Primary Care*. Oxford: Oxford University Press.

Kai, J., Bridgewater, R. and Spencer, J. (2001a) 'Just think of TB and Asians, that's all I ever hear': medical learners' views about training to work in an ethnically diverse society, *Medical Education*, 35: 250–6.

Kai, J., Spencer, J. and Woodward, N. (2001b) Wrestling with ethnic diversity: toward empowering educators, *Medical Education*, 35: 262–71.

Kalsi, S. (1996) Change and continuity in the funeral rituals of Sikhs in Britain, in G. Howarth and P. Jupp (eds) *Contemporary Issues in the Sociology of Death, Dying and Disposal*. Basingstoke: Macmillan.

Kaptchuk, T. and Eisenberg, D. (1998) The persuasive appeal of alternative medicine, *Annals Internal Medicine*, 129: 1061–5.

Karim, K., Bailey, M. and Tunna, K. (2000) Non-white ethnicity and the provision of specialist palliative care services: factors affecting doctors' referral patterns, *Palliative Medicine*, 14: 471–8.

Katz, J.S. (2000) Jewish perspective on death, dying and bereavement, in D. Dickenson, M. Johnson and J. Katz, *Death, Dying and Bereavement*. Sage Publications.

Kaur, J.S. (1996) The potential impact of cancer survivors on Native American cancer prevention and treatment, *Cancer Supplement*, 78:1578–81.

Kearney, M. (1997) *Mortally Wounded, Stories of Soul, Pain, Death and Healing*. New York: Touchstone.

Kelly, P. (2004) Cancer risk assessment, in R. Moore and D. Spiegel (eds) *Cancer, Culture and Communication*. New York: Kluwer Academic.

Kelly, W. and Trleson, S.R. (1950) Do cancer patients want to be told? *Surgery*, 27: 822.

Kelner, M. and Wellman, B. (1997) Health care and consumer choice: medical and alternative therapies, *Social Science and Medicine*, 45: 203–12.

Kernohan, E.E. (1996) Evaluation of a pilot study for breast and cervical cancer screening with Bradford's minority ethnic women; a community development approach, 1991–93, *British Journal of Cancer*, 29: S42–6.

Kierkegaard, S. (1944) *Kierkegaard Concluding Unscientific Postscript*. Translated by F. Swenson Princeton New Jersey. Prints at University Press for American Scandinavian Foundation.

Kittler, P. and Sucher, K. (1998) *Food and Culture in America: A Nutrition Handbook*. Belmont, CA: West/ Wadsworth.

Kleinman, A. (1970) Depression, somatization and the 'new cross cultural psychiatry', *Social Science and Medicine*, 11: 3–10.

Kleinman, A. (1980) *Patients and Healers in the Context of Culture*. Berkeley, CA: University of California Press.

Kleinman, A. (1990) *The Illness Narratives: Suffering, Healing and the Human Condition*. New York: Basic Books.

Kleinman, A. (1997) *Social Suffering*. Berkeley, CA: University of California Press.

Kleinman, A. (1998) *Experience and Its Moral Codes: Culture, Human Conditions and Disorder*. The Tanner Lectures on Human Values delivered at Stanford University.

Kleinman, A. and Kleinman, J. (1985) Somatisation, in A. Kleinman and B. Good (eds) Culture and Depression. Berkeley, CA: University of California.

Klonoff, E.A. and Landrine, H. (1994) Culture and gender diversity in common sense beliefs about the causes of six illnesses, *Journal of Behavioural Medicine*, 17: 407–18.

Koffman, J., Higginson, I. and Donaldson, N. (2003) Symptoms, severity in advanced cancer, assessed in two ethnic groups by interviewing, *Journal of the Royal Society of Medicine*, 96: 10–16.

Krause, I.B. (1989) Sinking heart, a Punjabi communication of distress, *Social Science and Medicine*, 29: 563–75.

Kuyken, W., Orley, J., Hudelson, P. and Sartorius, N. (1994) Quality-of-life assessment across cultures, *International Journal of Mental Health*, 23: 5–27.

Kvale, S. (1992) Postmodern psychology: a contradiction in terms, in S. Kvale (ed.) *Psychology and Postmodernism*. London: Sage.

La Borde, P. (2004) Vietnamese: Cultural Profile. EthnoMed, University of Washington, Seattle. http://ethnomed.org/ethnomed/cultures/vietnamese/vietnamese_cp.html#interpersonal

Lambert, H. and McKevitt, C. (2002) Anthropology in health research: from qualitative methods to multidisciplinarity, *British Medical Journal* 325: 210–13.

Landy, D. (1977) in D. Landy (ed.) *Culture, Disease and Healing: Studies in Medical Anthropology*. London: Macmillan.

Lannin, D.R., Matthews, H.F., Mitchell, J. *et al.* (2002) Impacting cultural attitudes in African-American women to decrease breast cancer mortality, *The American Journal of Surgery*, 184: 418–23.

Laubmeier, K., Zakowski, S. and Bair, J. (2004) The role of spirituality in the psychological adjustment to cancer: a test of the transactional model of stress and coping, *International Journal of Behavioural Medicine*, 11(1): 48–55.

Lauver, D. and Ho, C.H. (1993) Explaining delay in care seeking for breast cancer symptoms, *Journal of Applied Social Psychology*, 23: 1806–25.

Lee, M.M., Lin, S.S., Wrensch, M.R., Adler, S.R. and Eisenberg, D. (2000) Alternative therapies used by women with breast cancer in four ethnic populations, *Journal of the National Cancer Institute*, 92: 42–7.

Lee, S. and Whitehead, D. (1998) *Survey on Complementary Therapies*. The Sara Lee Trust: St Michael's Trust East Sussex. Unpublished.

Lee, A. and Wu, H. (2002) Diagnosis disclosure in cancer patients – when the family says 'No!', *Singapore Medical Journal*, 43(10): 533–8.

Lerner, I.J. (1984) The whys of cancer quackery, *Cancer*, 53(3) suppl: 815–19.

Levi Strauss, C. (1958) *Structural Anthropology*. Allen Lane. The Penguin Press.

Li, C.I., Malone, K.E. and Daling, J.R. (2003) Differences in breast cancer stage, treatment, and survival by race and ethnicity, *Archive of Internal Medicine*, 163: 49–56.

Little, D. (2001) *Breast Cancer in Asian Women*. EthnoMed. http://ethnomed.org/ethnomed/clin_topics/asian_br_cancer.html

Littlewood, R. and Dein, S. (2000) Introduction, in *Cultural Psychiatry and Medical Anthropology: An Introduction and a Reader*. London: Athlone.

Loehrer, S.R., Greger, H.A. and Weinberger, M. (1991) Knowledge and beliefs about cancer in a socioeconomically disadvantaged population, *Cancer*, 68: 1665–71.

Long, E. (1993) Breast cancer in African American women: review of the literature, *Cancer Nursing*, 16: 1–24.

Lopez, A. (1990) Causes of death: an assessment of global patterns of mortality around 1985, *World Health Statistics Quarterly*, 43: 91–104.

Lowe, R., Sheetal, C., Nasci, K. *et al.* (2001) Effect of ethnicity on denial of authorisation for emergency department care by managed gate keepers, *Academic Emergency Medicine*, 8(3): 259–66.

Luke, K. (1996) Cervical cancer screening: meeting the needs of minority ethnic women, *British Journal of Cancer Supplement*, 29: S27–50.

Lupton, D. (2004) *Medicine as Culture: Illness, Disease and the Body in Western Societies*. London: Sage Publications.

Lutz, C. (1988) *Unnatural Emotions: Everyday sentiments on a Micronesian Atoll and their Challenge to Western Theory*. Chicago, Il: University of Chicago Press.

McCaffery, K., Forrest, S., Waller, J. *et al.* (2003) Attitudes towards HPV testing: a qualitative study of beliefs among Indian, Pakistani, Afro Caribbean and White British women in the UK, *British Journal of Cancer*, 88(1): 42–6.

McCain, C., Rosenfeld, B. and Breitbart, W. (2003) Effect of spiritual well-being on end-of-life despair in terminally-ill cancer patients, *Lancet*, 361: 1603–7.

McCord, C. and Freeman, H.P. (1990) Excess mortality in Harlem, *New England Journal of Medicine*, 222: 173–7.

McCormack, V.A., Mangtani, P., Bhakta, D. *et al.* (2004) Heterogeneity of breast cancer risk within the South Asian female population in England: a population-based case-control study of first-generation migrants, *British Journal of Cancer*, 901: 160–6.

McEwen, B. and Wingfield, J. (2003) The concept of allostasis in biology and biomedicine, *Hormonal Behaviour*, 43(1): 2–15.

McGinnis, J. and Foege, W. (1993) Actual causes of death in the United States, *Journal of American Medical Association*, 270(18): 2207–12.

McKeown, T. (1979) *The Role of Medicine: Dream, Mirage or Nemesis*. Princeton, NJ: Princeton University Press.

Macbeth, H. (2001) Defining the ethnic group: important and impossible, in H. Macbeth and P. Shetty (eds) *Health and Ethnicity*. London: Taylor & Francis.

MacDowell, M., Guo, L. and Short, A. (2002) Preventive health services use, lifestyle behaviour risks, and self reported health status of women in Ohio by ethnicity and completed education status, *Women's Health Issues*, 12(2): 96–102.

Machiavelli, M., Leone, B., Romero, A. *et al.* (1989) Relation between delay and survival in 596 patients with breast cancer, *Oncology*, 46: 78–82.

Maclennan, A.H., Wilson, D.H. and Taylor, A.W. (1996) Prevalence and cost of alternative medicine in Australia, *Lancet*, 347: 569–73.

Malik, I. and Qureshi, A. (1997) Communication with cancer patients. Experiences in Pakistan, *Annals of the New York Academy of Sciences*, 809: 300–8.

Malinowski, B. (1935) *Coral Gardens and their Magic*. London: Allen and Unwin.

Margolis, M. (2003) Racial differences pertaining to a belief about lung cancer surgery, *Annals of Internal Medicine*, 139: 558–63.

Mariotto, A., Gigli, A., Caposaccia, R. *et al.* (2002) *SEERr Cancer Statistics Review 1973–1999: Complete Unlimited Duration Cancer Prevalence Estimates*. Bethesta, MD: National Cancer Institute.

Markus, H.R. and Kitayama, S. (1991) Culture and self: implications for cognition, emotion and motivation, *Psychological Review*, 98: 224–53.

Marsella, A., Sartorius, N., Jablensky, A. and Fenton, F. (1985) Cross cultural studies of depressive disorders: an overview, in A. Kleinman and B. Good (eds) *Culture and Depression*. Berkeley, CA: University of California.

Mason, S., Hussain-Gambles, M., Leese, B. *et al.* (2003) Representation of South Asian people in randomised clinical trials: analysis of trials, *British Medical Journal*, 326: 1244–5.

Massie, M., Gagnon, P. and Holland, J. (1994) Depression and suicide in patients with cancer, *Journal of Pain and Symptom Management*, 9(5): 325–40.

Matthews, H., Lanin, D. and Mitchell, J. (1994) Coming to terms with advanced breast cancer: Black women's narratives from Eastern North Carolina, *Social Science and Medicine*, 38: 789–800.

Merrill, R., Merrill, A. and Mayer, L. (2000) Factors associated with no surgery or radiation therapy for invasive cervical cancer in Black and White Women, *Ethnicity and Disease*, 10: 248–56.

Meyerowitz, B.E., Richardson, J., Hudson, S. and Leedham, B. (1998) Ethnicity and cancer outcomes; behavioural and psychosocial considerations, *Psychological Bulletin*, 123: 47–70.

Meyza, J. (1997) Truth-telling, information, communication with cancer patients in Poland, *Annals of the New York Academy of Science*, 809: 68–79.

Mickley, J., Soeken, K. and Belcher, A. (1992) Spiritual well-being, religiousness and hope among women with breast cancer, *Image: Journal of Nursing Scholarship*, 244: 267–72.

Millon-Underwood, S., Sanders, E. and Davis, M. (1993) Determinants of participation in state of the art cancer prevention, early detection/screening and treatment trials among African Americans, *Cancer Nursing*, 161: 25–33.

Mills, R. and Bhandari, S. (2003) *Health Insurance Coverage in the United States 2002*. Washington, DC: US Government Printing Office.

Miyaji, N. (1993) The power of compassion: truth telling among American doctors in the care of dying patients, *Social Science and Medicine*, 36: 249–64.

Mo, B. (1992) Modesty, sexuality and breast health in Chinese-American women, *Western Journal of Medicine*, 157: 260–4.

Montbriand, M.J. (1994) An overview of alternate therapies chosen by patients with cancer, *Oncology Nursing Forum*, 21: 1547–54.

Montbriand, M.J. (1997) Abandoned by medicine for alternative therapies: oncology patients' stories, *Cancer Nursing*, 21: 36–45.

Moore, R. and Butow, P. (2004) Culture and oncology: impact of context effects, in R. Moore and D. Spiegel (eds) *Cancer, Culture and Communication*. New York: Kluwer Academic/Plenum Publishers.

Moore, R. and Spiegel, D. (2004) *Cancer, Culture and Communication*. New York: Kluwer Academic/Plenum Publishers.

Morgan, C., Park, E. and Cortes, D. (1995) Beliefs, knowledge and behaviour about cancer among urban Hispanic women. *Journal of National Cancer Institute Monographs*, 18: 57–63.

Morris, B. (1994) *Anthropology of the Self: The Individual in Cultural Perspective*. London: Pluto Press.

Mumford, D.B. (1993) Somatisation: a transcultural perspective, *International Review of Psychiatry*, 5: 231–42.

Musick, M.A., Koenig, H.G., Hays, J.C. and Cohen, H.J. (1998) Religious activity and depression among community-dwelling elderly persons with cancer – the modelling effect of race, *Journal of Gerontology Social Sciences*, 53: S218–227.

Mystakidou, K., Liossi, C., Vlachos, L. and Papadimitriou, J. (1996) Disclosure of diagnostic information to cancer patients in Greece, *Palliative Medicine*, 103: 195–200.

Naish, J., Browner, J. and Denton, B. (1994) Intercultural consultations: investigation of the factors that deter non-English speaking women from attending their GPs for cervical screening, *British Medical Journal*, 309: 1126–8.

Narikiyo, T.A. and Kameoka, V.A. (1992) Attributions of mental illness and judgments about help seeking among Japanese-American and white American students, *Journal of Counseling Psychology*, 39: 363–9.

Nazroo, J. and Davey-Smith, G. (2001) The contribution of socio-economic position to health differentials between ethnic groups. Evidence from the United States and Britain, in H. Macbeth and P. Shetty (eds) *Health and Ethnicity*. London: Taylor & Francis.

NCI (2002) Cancer Screening Overview. *Scientific basis for cancer screening*. National Cancer Institute. Available: Cancer.Gov.

Neighbors, H. (1987) Barriers to medical care among adult blacks: What happens to the uninsured? *Journal of National Medical Association*, 79: 489–92.

Neighbors, H.W., Musick, M.A. and Williams, D.R. (1998) The African American minister as a source of help for serious personal crises: bridge or barrier to mental health care? *Health Education and Behaviour*, 25: 759–77.

Nelson, K., Geiger, A.M. and Mangione, C.M. (2002) Effect of health beliefs on delays in care for abnormal cervical cytology in a multiethnic population, *Journal of General Internal Medicine*, 17: 709–16.

Nelson, C.J., Rosenfeld, B., Breitbart, W. *et al.* (2002) Spirituality, religion, and depression in the terminally ill, *Psychosomatics*, 43(3): 213–20.

Nemeek, M. (1990) Health beliefs and breast examination among black women, *Health Values*, 14: 41–52.

Neuberger, J. (1987) *Caring for Dying People of Different Faiths*. London: Austin Cornish & Lisa Sainsbury Foundations.

Neuberger, J. (1998) Cultural issues in palliative care, in G. Doyle, W. Hanks and N. MacDonald (eds) *The Oxford Textbook of Palliative Medicine*. Oxford: Oxford University Press.

Neuberger, J. (2004) *Caring for Dying People of Different Faiths*, 3rd edn. London: Mosby.

Ngo-Metzger, Q., Mccarthy, E., Burns, R. *et al.* (2003) Older Asian Americans and Pacific Islanders dying of cancer use hospice less frequently than older white patients, *American Journal of Medicine*, 115: 47–53.

Nielsen, B., MacMillan, S. and Diaz, E. (1992) Instruments that measure beliefs about cancer from a cultural perspective, *Cancer Nursing*, 15(2): 109–15.

Nobels, W.W. (1991) African philosophy. Foundation for black psychology, in R.L. Jones (ed.) *Black Psychology*. Berkeley, CA: Cobb and Henry.

Novack, D.H., Plumer, R., Smith, R.L. *et al.* (1979) Changes in physicians' attitudes towards telling the cancer patient, *Journal of the American Medical Association*, 241: 897–900.

Office for National Statistics (2002) *Mortality Statistics: Cause. England and Wales*. London: TSO.

Oken, D. (1961) 'What to tell cancer patients'. A study of medical attitudes, *Journal of the American Medical Association*, 175: 1120–8.

Paice, J. and O'Donnell, J. (2004) Cultural experience of cancer pain, in R. Moore and D. Spiegel (eds) *Cancer, Culture and Communication*. New York: Kluwer Academic/Plenum Publishers.

Papadopoulos, I. (2001) Let's Talk About Cancer: An exploration of the impact of culture on cancer attitudes and related practices of Greek and Greek Cypriots living in North London. London: Greek and Greek Cypriot Community of Enfield and Middlesex University.

Pargament, K. (1997) *The Psychology of Religion and Coping*. New York: Guilford.

Parker, R. and Hopwood, P. (2000) *Literature Review: Quality of Life of Black and Ethnic Minority Groups with Cancer*. Cancer Research UK Psychological Medicine Group. Manchester: University of Manchester.

Parkin, D. (2001) Ethnicity and the risk of cancer, in H. Macbeth and P. Shetty (eds) *Health and Ethnicity*. London: Taylor and Francis.

Parkin, D.M., Lara, D. and Muir, C.S. (1988) Estimates of the world wide frequency of sixteen major cancers, *International Journal of Cancer*, 41: 184–97.

Patterson, J. (1987) *The Dread Disease: Cancer and Modern American Culture*. Cambridge, MA: Harvard University Press.

Pederson, L., Ahluwalia, J., Harris, K. *et al.* (2000) Smoking cessation among African Americans: what we know and do not know about intervention and self-quitting, *Preventive Medicine*, 31(1): 23–38.

Pellegrino, E. (1998) Emerging ethical issues in palliative care, *Journal of American Medical Association*, 279(19): 1521.

Pena, D., Munoz, C. and Grumbach, K. (2003) Cross-cultural education in US medical schools: development of an assessment tool, *Academic Medicine*, 78: 615–22.

Perez-Sable, E.J., Sabogal, F., Otero-Sabogal, R. *et al.* (1992) Misconceptions about cancer among Latinos and Anglos, *Journal of the American Medical Association*, 272: 31–2.

Peters-Golden, H. (1982) Breast cancer: varied perceptions of social support in the illness experience, *Social Science and Medicine*, 16: 483–91.

Peto, R., Darby, S., Deo, H. *et al.* (2000) Smoking, smoking cessation and lung cancer: a combination of national statistics and two case controlled studies, *British Medical Journal*, 321: 2323–9.

Pham, C.T. and McPhee, S.J. (1992) Knowledge, attitudes, and practices of breast and cervical cancer screening among Vietnamese women, *Journal of Cancer Education*, 74: 305–10.

Phipps, E., True, G., Harris, D., Chong, U. *et al.* (2003) Approaching the end of life: attitudes, preferences and behaviours of African American and white patients and their family care givers, *Journal of Clinical Oncology*, 213: 549–54.

Pill, R. and Stot, N. (1982) Concepts of illness – causation and responsibility: some preliminary data from a sample of working class mothers, *Social Science and Medicine*, 16: 43–52.

Polednak, A.P. (1986) Breast cancer in black and white women in New York State. Case distribution and incidence rates by clinical stage at diagnosis, *Cancer*, 58: 807–15.

Pooransingh, S. and Ramaiah, S. (2001) Smoking amongst South Asians in the United Kingdom [electronic response to H. Barratt, UK governance launches anti-tobacco campaign for Asians].

Powe, B. (1995a) Fatalism among the elderly African Americans: effects on colon rectal screening, *Cancer Nursing*, 18: 385–92.

Powe, B. (1995) Perceptions of cancer fatalism among African Americans: the influence of education, income and cancer knowledge, *Journal of National Black Nurses Association*, 72: 41–8.

Powe, B. (1996) Cancer fatalism among African Americans: review of the literature, *Nursing Outlook*, 441: 18–21.

Powe, B. (1997) Cancer fatalism: spiritual perspective, *Journal of Religion and Health*, 362: 135–44.

Powe, B. (2002) Promoting faecal occult blood testing in rural African American Women, *Cancer Practice*, 103: 139–46.

Powe, B. (2003) Cancer fatalism: the state of the science, *Cancer Nursing*, 262: 454–65.

Powe, B. and Johnson, A. (1995) Fatalism among African Americans, Philosophical Perspective, *Journal of Religion and Health*, 34: 119–25.

Powe, B. and Weinrich, S. (1999) An intervention to decrease cancer fatalism among rural elders, *Oncology Nursing Forum*, 263: 583–8.

Price, J.H., Desmond, S.M., Wallace, M. *et al.* (1998) Differences in black and white adolescents' perceptions about cancer, *Journal of School Health*, 58: 66–70.

Proctor, B.D. and Dalaker, J. (2002) *Poverty in the United States: 2001*. Washington, DC: US Government Printing Office. US Census Bureau Current Population Reports.

Pruyn, J.F., Rijckman, R.M., van Brunschot, C. *et al.* (1985) Cancer patients' personality and characteristics, physician-patient communication and adoption of morman diet, *Social Science & Medicine*, 20: 831–47.

Puchalski, C. (1999) Taking a spiritual history allows clinicians to understand patients more fully. An interview with Dr Christiana Puchalski, by A.L. Romer, *Innovations in End of Life Care*, 1: 6.

Rachels, J. (2002) The challenge of cultural relativism in *Elements of Moral Philosophy*. Maidenhead: Mc Graw-Hill.

Raleigh, E. (1992) Sources of hope in chronic illness, *Oncology Nursing Forum*, 19: 443–8.

Ralston, J.D., Taylor, V.M., Yasui, Y. *et al.* (2003) Knowledge of cervical cancer risk factors among Chinese immigrants in Seattle, *Community Health*, 281: 41–57.

Ramakrishna, J. and Weiss, M. (1992) Health, illness and immigration. East Indians in the United States, *Western Journal of Medicine*, 157(3): 265–70.

Ramirez, A.J., Bogdanovic, M.R. and Jasovicgasic, M. (1991) Psychosocial adjustment to cancer – cultural considerations, *European Journal of Psychiatry*, 5: 9–18.

Ramirez, A.J., Westcombe, A.M., Burgess, C.C. *et al.* (1999) Factors predicting delayed presentation of symptomatic breast cancer. A systematic review, *The Lancet*, 353: 1127–31.

Rees, W. (1986) Immigrants and the hospice, *Health Trends*, 18: 89–91.

Reese, D. and Ahern, R. (1999) Hospice access and use by African-Americans: addressing cultural and institutional barriers through participatory action research, *Social Work*, 44(6): 549–60.

Rice, M. (1987) Inner-city hospital closures/relocations: race, income, status and legal issues, *Social Science and Medicine*, 24: 889–96.

Rider, I. (1997) Gynaecological investigations and surgery, in G. Andrews (ed.) *Women's Health Issues*. London: Baillière Tindall.

Ries, L., Eisner, M., Kosary, C. *et al.* (2003) *SEER Cancer Statistics Review 1975–2000.* Bethesda, MD: National Cancer Institute.

Ries, L., Eisner, M., Kosary, C. *et al.* (2004) *SEER Cancer Statistics Review 1975–2001.* Bethesda, MD: National Cancer Institute.

Roberts, J.A., Brown, D., Elkins, T. and Larson, D.B. (1997) Factors influencing views of patients with gynaecologic cancer about end of life decisions, *American Journal of Obstetrics and Gynaecology*, 176: 166–72.

Roberts, C. and Manchester, K. (2001) *The Archaeology of Disease.* Bradford: Sutton Publishing.

Rosenblatt, P. (1997) Grief in small scale societies, in M. Parkes, P. Languani and M. Young (eds) *Death and Bereavement Across Cultures.* London: Routledge.

Russell, R. (2002) Beta-carotene and lung cancer, *Pure Applied Chemistry*, 74(8): 1461–7.

Rutledge, E. (2001) The struggle for equality in healthcare continues, *Journal of Healthcare Management*, 465: 313–26.

Saxena, S. (1994) Quality of life assessment in cancer patients in India: cross cultural issues, in J. Orley and W. Kewken (eds) *Quality of Life Assessment: International Perspective.* Heidelberg: Springer-Verlag.

Scheff, T. (1979) *Catharsis in Healing, Ritual and Drama.* Berkeley, CA: University of California Press.

Schumaker, J.D. (2004) *Hospice Care in the United States.* http://www.bbriefings.com/pdf/886/lth041_r_schumacher.pdf

Seale, C. (1998) *Constructing Death: the Sociology of Death and Bereavement.* Cambridge: Cambridge University Press.

Seale, C., Addington-Hall, J. and McCarthy, M. (1997) Awareness of dying: prevalence, causes and consequences, *Social Science and Medicine*, 45: 477–84.

Seers, K. and Carroll, D. (1998) Relaxation techniques for acute pain management: a systematic review, *Journal of Advanced Nursing*, 27: 466–75.

Sen, M. (1997) Communication with cancer patients: the influence of age, gender, education and health insurance status, in A. Surbone and M. Zwitter (eds) *Communication with the Cancer Patient. Information and Truth.* New York: The New York Academy of Sciences.

Senior, P. and Bhopal, R. (1994) Ethnicity as a variable in epidemiological research, *British Medical Journal*, 309: 327–30.

Sensky, T. (1996) Enlisting lay beliefs across cultures: principles and methodology, *British Journal of Cancer Supplement*, 29: S63–65.

Sharma, U. (1990) Using alternative therapies: marginal medicine and central concerns, in P. Abbott and G. Payne (ed.) *New Directions in the Sociology of Health.* Falmer Press.

Shavers, V. and Brown, M. (2002) Racial and ethnic disparities in the receipt of cancer treatment, *Journal of the National Cancer Institute*, 94: 334–57.

Shavers, V., Brown, M., Potosky, A. and Carnie, N. (2004) Race/ethnicity on the receipt of Watchful Waiting for initial management of prostate cancer. *Journal of General Internal Medicine*, 19: 146–55.

Shumay, D.M., Maskarinec, G., Gotay, C.C. *et al.* (2002) Determinants of the degree of complimentary and alternative medicine use among patients with cancer, *Journal of Alternative and Complimentary Medicine*, 8: 661–71.

Shuster, E. (1997) Fifty years later: the significance of the Nuremberg Code, *New England Journal of Medicine*, 337: 1436–40.

Siahpush, M. (1998) Post modern values, dissatisfaction with conventional medicine and popularity of alternative therapies, *Journal of Sociology*, 34: 58–70.

Siegel, B. (1993) *Love, Medicine, Miracles*. New York: Harper Collins.

Sikora, K. (1997) Complementary medicine in cancer, *Cancer Care*, 9–11.

Silveira, E. and Ebrahim, S. (1995) Mental health and health status of elderly Bengalis and Somalis in London, *Age and Aging*, 24: 474–80.

Simmonds, R., Sque, M., Goddard, J. *et al.* (2001) Improving access to palliative care services for ethnic minority groups. A report of the study carried out by St Catherine's Palliative Care Centre, funded by the National Lottery community fund in 2001.

Simonton, O.C., Mathews-Simonton, S. and Sparks, T. (1980) Psychological intervention in the treatment of cancer, *Psychosomatics*, 21: 226–33.

Singer, M. and Baer, M. (1995) *Critical Medical Anthropology*. Amityville, NY: Baywood Press.

Singh, G., Miller, B., Hankey, B. and Edwards, B. (2003) Area socioeconomic variations in US cancer incidence, mortality stage, treatment and survival 1975–1999. Bethesda MD, National Cancer Institute. *NCI Cancer Surveillance Monograph Series*. Number 4. NIH Publication No. 03–5417.

Skultans, V. (1998) Anthropology and narrative, in T. Greenlahalgh and B. Hurwitz (eds) *Narrative Based Medicine: Dialogue and Discourse in Clinical Practice*. London: British Medical Journal Books.

Slevin, M., Stubbs, L., Plant, H. and Wilson, P. (1990) Attitudes to chemotherapy – comparing views of patients with cancer with those doctors, nurses and the general public, *British Medical Journal*, 300: 1458–60.

Smaje, C. (1995) *Health, Race and Ethnicity*. London: Kings Fund Institute.

Smaje, C. and Field, D. (1997) Absent minorities? Ethnicity and the use of palliative care services, in D. Field, J. Hockey and N. Small (eds) *Death, Gender and Ethnicity*. London: Routledge.

Smedley, B.D., Stith, A. and Nelson, A.R.l. (2002) *Unequal Treatment: Confronting Racial and Ethnic Disparities in Health Care*. Washington, DC: National Academic Press.

Snow, L.F. (1983) Traditional health beliefs and practices among lower class black Americans, *Western Journal of Medicine*, 139: 820–9.

Sontag, S. (1989) *Illness as a Metaphor: AIDS ands its Metaphors*. New York: Anglia.

Souhami, R. and Tobias, R. (2002) *Cancer and Its Management*, 4th edn. Oxford: Blackwell.

Spencer, S.M., Lehman, J.M., Wynings, C., Arena, P. *et al.* (1999) Concerns about breast cancer in relation to psychological well-being in a multi-ethnic sample of early stage patents, *Health Psychology*, 18: 159–68.

Spiegel, E., Bloom, J. K., Kraemer, H. C. *et al.* (1989) Effects of psychosocial treatment on patients with metastatic breast cancer, *Lancet*, 2: 888–91.

Spiegel, D., Morrow, G.R., Classen, C. *et al.* (1999) Group psychotherapy for recently diagnosed breast cancer patients: a multicenter feasibility study, *Psycho-Oncology*, 8: 482–93.

Spruyt, O. (1999) Community-based palliative care for Bangladeshi patients in east London: accounts of bereaved carers, *Palliative Medicine*, 13: 110–29.

Stacey, J. (1997) *Teratologies: A Cultural Study of Cancer*. London: Routledge.

Stjernsward, J. and Clark, D. (2003) Palliative medicine – a global perspective, in D. Doyle, G. Hanks, N. Cherny and K. Calman (eds) *Oxford Textbook of Palliative Medicine*. Oxford: Oxford University Press.

Stoll, B. (1996) Obesity, social class and Western diet: a link to breast cancer prognosis, *European Journal of Cancer*, 32: 1293–5.

Stoll, B. (2000) Affluence, obesity and breast cancer, *Breast Journal*, (6)2: 146–9.

Stoller, P. (2004) *Stranger in the Village of the Sick: A Memoir of Cancer, Sorcery and Healing*. Boston: Beacon Press.

Straughan, P. and Seow, A. (1998) Fatalism re-conceptualised: the concept to predict health screening behaviour. *Journal of Gender, Culture and Health*, 32: 85–100.

Surbone, A. and Zwitter, M. (1997) Communication with the cancer patient: information and truth, *Annals of the New York Academy of Science*, 809.

Sussman, L.K., Robins, L.N. and Earls, F. (1987) Treatment-seeking for depression by black and white Americans, *Social Science and Medicine*, 24: 187–96.

Sutton, S., Bickler, G. and Sancho-Aldridge, J. (1994) Prospective study of predictors of attendance of breast screening in inner London, *Journal of Epidemiology & Community Health*, 48: 65–73.

Swanson, G.M. and Bailar, J.C. 3rd (2002) Selection and description of cancer clinical trials participants--science or happenstance? *Cancer*, 95: 950–9.

Taussig, M. (1980) *The Devil and Commodity Fetishism*. Chapel Hill: University of North Carolina Press.

Taylor, K. (1988) 'Telling bad news': physicians and the disclosure of undesirable information, *Sociology of Health and Illness*, 10: 100–33.

Taylor, E., Outlaw, F., Bernado, T. *et al.* (1999) Spiritual conflicts associated with praying about cancer, *Psychooncology*, 8(5): 386–94.

Thomas, K., Carr, J., Westlake, L. and Williams, B. (1991) Use of unorthodox and conventional health care in Great Britain, *British Medical Journal*, 302: 207–10.

Thomas, S. and Kearsley, J. (1993) Betel quid and oral cancer: a review, *European Journal of Cancer. Part B, Oral Oncology*, 29B: 251–5.

Turner, V. (1969) *The Ritual Process: Structure and Anti-structure*. Chicago: Aldine.

Uba, L. (1992) *Cultural Barriers to Health Care for Southeast Asian Refugees*, *Public Health Report*, vol. 107 September/October 1992, pp. 544–8.

US Bureau of the Census, *Census 2000*, Redistricting Data.

US Department of Health and Human Services (1998) *Tobacco Use Among US Racial/Ethnic Minority Groups- African Americans, American Indians, and Alaska Natives, Asian Americans, and Pacific Islanders, and Hispanics. A report for the Surgeon General*. Atlanta, GA: US Department of Health and Human Services, Centers for Disease Control and Prevention. National Center for Chronic Disease Prevention and Health Promotion, Office on Smoking and Health.

US Department of Health and Human Services (2000) *Healthy People 2010: Understanding and Improving Health*. Washington, DC: US Government Printing Office.

Uskul, A. (2001) Department of Psychology, Graduate Program, York University. *Cultural Determinants of Medical Help Seeking for Symptoms of Breast Cancer*. http://www.cehip.org/menujs.html

Van Gennep, A. (1966) *The Rites of Passage*. Chicago: The University of Chicago Press.

Van Ryn, M. and Burke, J. (2000) The effect of patient race and socioeconomic status on physicians perceptions of patients, *Social Science and Medicine*, 50: 813–28.

Velikova, G., Booth, L., Johnston, C. and Forman, D. (2004) Breast cancer outcomes in South Asian population of West Yorkshire, *British Journal of Cancer*, 90: 1926–32.

Vermeire, E., Hearnshaw, H., Van Royen, P. and Denekens, J. I. (2001) Patients adherence to treatment: three decades of research. A comprehensive review, *Journal of Clinical Pharmacological Therapy*, 265: 331–42.

Vernon, S.W., Vogel, V.G., Halabi, S., Jackson, G. *et al.* (1992) Breast cancer screening behaviours and attitudes in three ethnic/racial groups, *Cancer*, 69: 165–74.

Waechter, E.H. (1971) Children's awareness of fatal illness, *American Journal of Nursing*, 7: 1168–672.

Ward, E., Jemal, A., Cokkinides, V., Singh, G.K. *et al.* (2004) Cancer disparities by race/ethnicity and socioeconomic status, *CA: A Cancer Journal for Clinicians*, 54: 78–93.

Weinstein, N. (1987) Unrealistic optimism about susceptibility to health problems: conclusions from a community-wide sample, *Journal of Behavioural Medicine*, 10: 481–500.

Weis, H.H., Bartsch, F., Hennies, M., Rietschel, M. *et al.* (1998) Complementary medicine in cancer patients: demand, patients attitudes and psychological beliefs, *Oncology*, 21: 144–9.

Weisburger, J. and Chung, F. (2002) Mechanisms of chronic disease causation by nutritional factors and tobacco products and their prevention by tea polyphenols, *Food and Chemical Toxicology*, 40: 1145–54.

Weisman, A. and Worden, J. (1977) The existential plight in cancer: significance of the first 100 days. *International Journal of Psychiatry in Medicine*, 7(1): 1–15.

Weiss, M. (2001) Cultural epidemiology. *Special Issue of Anthropology and Medicine*, 8(1).

WHO (1986) *Ottowa Charter for Health Promotion*. Geneva: WHO.

WHOQOL Group (1993) Study protocol for the World Health Organisation project to develop a Quality of Life measurement instrument (the WHOQOL), *Quality of Life Research*, 2: 153–9.

Wiencke, J. (2004) Impact of race/ethnicity on molecular pathways in human cancer, *National Review of Cancer*, 4(1): 79–84.

Wigodor, G. (1966) Shiva in *The Encyclopaedia of Jewish Religion*. R. Zwiwerblossky (ed.). New York: Holt, Reinhert & Winston inclusive.

Wilkinson, S., Gomella, L.G., Smith, J.A. *et al.* (2002) Attitudes in use of complementary medicine in men with prostate cancer, *Journal of Urology*, 168: 2505–9.

Witte, K. and Allen, M. (2000) A meta-analysis of fear appeals: implications for effective public health campaigns, *Health Education and Behaviour*, 27: 501–15.

Wood, S., Friedland, B. and McGory, C. (2001) *Informed Consent: From Good Intention to Sound Practices*. New York: Population Council.

World Health Organisation (1991) *World Health Statistics Annual 1990*. Geneva: World Health Organisation.

World Health Organisation (1999) *World Health Report: Making A Difference*. Geneva: World Health Organisation.

World Health Organisation (2002) *Cancer Pain Relief and Palliative Care*. Geneva: World Health Organisation.

World Medical Association (2000) *Declaration of Helsinki*. http://www.wma.net/e/policy/b3.htm

Yee, L. (1997) *Breaking Barriers: Towards Culturally Competent General Practice*. London: Royal College of General Practitioners.

Younge, D., Moreau, P., Ezzat, A. and Gray, A. (1997) Communicating with cancer patients in Saudi Arabia, in A. Surbonne and M. Zwitter (eds) *Communication with the Cancer Patient: Information and Truth*, Annals of the New York Academy of Sciences. Vol.809. New York: The New York Academy of Sciences.

Zacharia, E. R., Pedersen, C., Jensen, A. and Ehrnrooth, E. (2003) Association of perceived physician communication style with patient satisfaction, distress, cancer related self-efficacy and perceived control over disease, *British Journal of Cancer*, 88(5): 658–65.

Zborowski, M. (1952) Cultural components in the response to pain, *Journal of Social Issues*, 8: 16–30.

Zola, I. (1966) Culture and symptoms: an analysis of patients' presenting complaints. *American Sociological Review*, 31: 615–30.

Index

LOSS, CHANGE AND BEREAVEMENT IN PALLIATIVE CARE

Pam Firth, Gill Luff and David Oliviere

- How do professionals meet the needs of bereaved people?
- How do professionals undertake best practice with individuals, groups, families and communities?
- What are the implications for employing research to influence practice?

This book provides a resource for working with a complex range of loss situations and includes chapters on childhood bereavement, and individual and family responses to loss and change. It contains the most up-to-date work in the field presented by experienced practitioners and researchers and is relevant not only for those working in specialist palliative care settings, but for professionals in general health and social care sectors.

Strong links are maintained between research and good practice throughout the book. These are reinforced by the coherent integration of international research material and the latest thinking about loss and bereavement. Experts and clinicians draw upon their knowledge and practice, whilst the essential perspective of the service user is central to this book.

Loss, Change and Bereavement in Palliative Care provides essential reading for a range of professional health and social care disciplines practising at postgraduate or post-registration/qualification level. It challenges readers, at an advanced level, on issues of loss, change and bereavement.

Contributors
Lesley Adshead, Jenny Altschuler, Peter Beresford, Grace H. Christ, Suzy Croft, Pam Firth, Shirley Firth, Richard Harding, Felicity Hearn, Jennie Lester, Gill Luff, Linda Machin, Jan McLaren, David Oliviere, Ann Quinn, Phyllis R. Silverman, Jean Walker, Karen Wilman.

Contents
Notes on the contributors – Series editor's preface – Acknowledgements – Foreword – Introduction – The context of loss, change and bereavement in palliative care – Mourning: a changing view – Research in practice – Illness and loss within the family – Life review with the terminally ill – Narrative therapies – The death of a child – Interventions with bereaved children – Involving service users in palliative care: from theory to practice – Excluded and vulnerable groups of service users – Carers: current research and developments – Groupwork in palliative care – Cultural perspectives on loss and bereavement – Conclusions – Index.

240pp   0 335 21323 5 (Paperback)   0 335 21324 3 (Hardback)

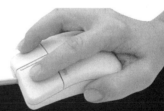
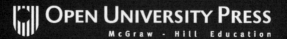